Epilepsy in childhood and adolescence
Third edition

Jhamara Athanda

Richard Appleton, MA, DCH, FRCP, FRCPCH
Consultant Paediatric Neurologist
The Roald Dahl EEG Unit
Department of Neurology
Royal Liverpool Children's NHS Trust (Alder Hey)
Liverpool, UK

John Gibbs, MD, DCH, MRCP, FRCPCH
Consultant Paediatrician
Children's Department
Countess of Chester Hospital NHS Trust
Chester, UK

MD Martin Dunitz
Taylor & Francis Group
LONDON AND NEW YORK

© 1995, 1998, 2004 Martin Dunitz, a member of the Taylor & Francis Group plc

First published in the United Kingdom in 1995
by Martin Dunitz, a member of the Taylor & Francis Group plc, 2 Park Square, Milton Park, Abingdon,
Oxfordshire OX14 4 RN

Tel.:   +44 (0)1235 828600
Fax.:   +44 (0)1235 829000
E-mail: info@dunitz.co.uk
Website: http://www.dunitz.co.uk

Reprinted 2004

Although every effort has been made to ensure that all owners of copyright material have been acknowledged in
this publication, we would be glad to acknowledge in subsequent reprints or editions any omissions brought to
our attention.

The Author has asserted his right under the Copyright, Designs and Patents Act 1988 to be identified as the
Author of this Work.

Although every effort has been made to ensure that drug doses and other information are presented accurately in
this publication, the ultimate responsibility rests with the prescribing physician. Neither the publishers nor the
authors can be held responsible for errors or for any consequences arising from the use of information contained
herein. For detailed prescribing information or instructions on the use of any product or procedure discussed
herein, please consult the prescribing information or instructional material issued by the manufacturer.

A CIP record for this book is available from the British Library.

ISBN 1 84184 362 8

Distributed in North and South America by
Taylor & Francis
2000 NW Corporate Blvd
Boca Raton, FL 33431, USA

Within Continental USA
Tel: 800 272 7737; Fax: 800 374 3401
Outside Continental USA
Tel: 561 994 0555; Fax: 561 361 6018
E-mail: orders@crcpress.com

Distributed in the rest of the world by
Thomson Publishing Services
Cheriton House
North Way
Andover, Hampshire SP10 5BE, UK
Tel.: +44 (0)1264 332424
E-mail: salesorder.tandf@thomsonpublishingservices.co.uk

Composition by Wearset Ltd, Boldon, Tyne and Wear

Printed and bound in Spain by Grafos SA

Contents

Acknowledgement

The authors are grateful to their families (particularly Jeanette and Hilary) for their patience and support and to Sandra Schofield, Pat McCarrick, Elma Ebben and Judith Baker for their understanding and assistance in the preparation of this third edition. Thankyou.

Preface

Within the past few years there has been a period of rapid expansion in our understanding of epilepsy. The discovery of an increasing number of gene mutations responsible for various types of epilepsy offers intriguing insights into not only the molecular, but also the genetic basis of epilepsy. The development of new anti-epileptic drugs and refinements to epilepsy surgery are widening the therapeutic options for epilepsy. In addition, the classification of the epilepsies continues to evolve based on an increased understanding of the molecular genetics of the condition, and this includes the recognition of possible novel epilepsy syndromes. The new edition of this book considers all of these exciting developments as well as addressing the essential features of the diagnosis, investigation, management and impact of epilepsy in childhood and adolescence.

Advances in our understanding of epilepsy would only be of limited benefit without concurrent improvements in the provision of epilepsy services. Fortunately, in the United Kingdom, there are several initiatives that are likely to enhance epilepsy services. The deficiencies in the provision of epilepsy care revealed by the National Sentinel Clinical Audit of Epilepsy-Related Death have provided a clear impetus for change. In addition, the National Service Framework for Children and guidance from the Scottish Intercollegiate Guidelines Network (SIGN) and National Institute for Clinical Excellence

(NICE) on both the general and specific drug management of epilepsy should lead to further improvements in epilepsy services. Nevertheless, considerable work is still required to ensure that these improvements become a reality.

Hopefully, this book will stimulate interest in epilepsy, provide a useful and practical knowledge base, offer a helpful summary of recent advances and assist readers in taking advantage of the current initiatives to provide more effective epilepsy services for children and adolescents.

Richard Appleton
John Gibbs

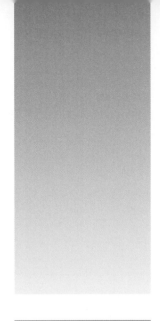

Introduction

Definitions

Seizures and epilepsy are clinical phenomena resulting from abnormal and excessive excitability of the cortical neurones of the cerebral hemispheres. They may be defined in both physiological and clinical terms:

Physiological

Epilepsy is the name for occasional sudden excessive rapid and local discharges of grey matter (Jackson, 1873)[1]

Clinical

An epileptic seizure is an intermittent, paroxysmal, stereotyped disturbance of consciousness, behaviour, emotion, motor function, perception or sensation (which may occur singly or in any combination) that on clinical grounds results from cortical neuronal discharge.

Epilepsy is a condition in which seizures recur, usually spontaneously

---

Although 'epilepsy' defines recurrent, largely unprovoked seizures, it is important to realize that an epileptic seizure may occur in non-epileptic patients subjected to a wide range of both direct cerebral and systemic insults *(Table 1)*. This is particularly common in children under the age of 5 years. Such provoked epileptic seizures should not be diagnosed as epilepsy.

Table 1
Cerebral and systemic insults that may result in epileptic seizures.

Fever	Renal failure	Drugs (e.g. alcohol abuse; solvents;
Hypoxia	Hepatic failure	Ecstasy)
Hypoglycaemia	Porphyria	Drug withdrawal
Hypocalcaemia		Toxins
Electrolyte imbalance		Trauma
Hypertension		
Inborn errors of metabolism		

An epileptic seizure always causes a disorganization or impairment of one or several brain functions; although these disturbances are usually clinically obvious, they may be subtle and not recognized.

The clinical event is accompanied by characteristic electro-encephalographic (EEG) changes of either a spike or sharp wave (the 'epileptic discharge'). These discharges may be local (focal) or diffuse (generalized). They may be recorded from the surface (scalp) EEG electrodes, but occasionally only from deeper (depth) electrodes. However, it must be realized that an epileptic discharge (spike or sharp wave) is not always accompanied by a clinical change. This emphasizes the point that epilepsy is a clinical, and not an EEG diagnosis.

The terms 'seizures', 'convulsions' and 'fits' are often used to mean the same thing (e.g. febrile seizure/convulsion/fit). The term 'convulsion' is used to define and differentiate an attack in which there are involuntary muscle contractions that are sustained (tonic), interrupted (clonic) or both (e.g. tonic–clonic or grand mal convulsion) from a seizure in which there is no abnormal muscle activity (e.g. an absence seizure). Most patients (and families of children) who have epilepsy tend to use the words 'fit' and 'convulsion' synonymously, and rarely spontaneously use the term seizure. More commonly, they may use words or terms such as, 'funny turns' or 'funny dos', 'twizzles' or 'shakes'.

Differences between childhood and adult epilepsy

In children, unlike in adults, many factors determine both whether epilepsy is likely to develop and the clinical and EEG manifestations of the seizures:

- Age
- Growth
- Development
- The 'environment'
- Genetic factors (as yet largely undetermined)

There are a number of significant differences between the occurrence, types and treatment of epilepsy in children and in adults *(Table 2)*.

Table 2
Differences between childhood and adult epilepsy.

Characteristics of epilepsy in children
1. Large differential diagnosis (see Chapter 1 on Diagnosis)

2. Heterogeneous condition — many epilepsy syndromes
         — many causes
         — many prognoses

3. The usual refractory seizure type is generalized (atonic, tonic or myoclonic) rather than partial
4. Most cases are idiopathic
5. Not a static condition (evolves and changes with age)
6. Not necessarily a life-long condition
7. Unclear but potentially important relationship between seizures (and their treatment with antiepileptic drugs) and learning/behavioural difficulties
8. Treatment must take account of educational issues and family dynamics
9. Need for consideration of the effects of antiepileptic drugs on the immature, developing brain

Epidemiology

Incidence

20–50 per 100 000 per year

Prevalence

4–10 per 1000 (active epilepsy)

There are no precise data on the prevalence of epilepsy in children. The figure of 0.7–0.8% of all school children (aged 5–17 years) is often quoted, and is similar to adult data. If this figure is accurate, and given the population of school-age children in England, Wales, Scotland and Northern Ireland to be 11.9 million (Office for National Statistics data 2001), this would indicate the total number of school children with epilepsy at any point in time to be approximately

85 000. This does not include pre-school children, and therefore the total number may possibly be closer to 90 or 95 000.

The lifetime cumulative incidence of epilepsy, derived from a large population-based study, is approximately 3% (*Figure 1*).[2,3] The discrepancy between lifetime cumulative incidence and prevalence reflects the transient nature of the condition in many patients.

Approximately one-third of all epilepsies that begin in childhood will have shown a (usually spontaneous) remission by puberty, which is then usually sustained throughout adult life.

Mortality

The standardized mortality ratio (SMR)

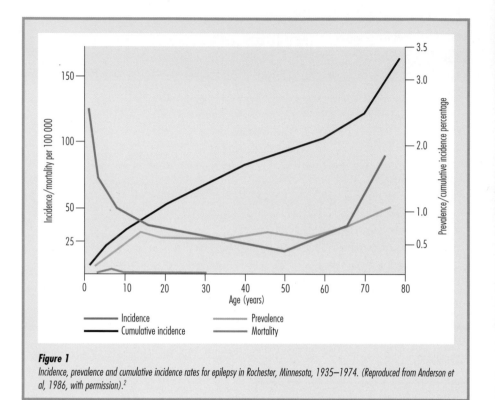

Figure 1
Incidence, prevalence and cumulative incidence rates for epilepsy in Rochester, Minnesota, 1935–1974. (Reproduced from Anderson et al, 1986, with permission).[2]

for epilepsy is high and approximately 2–3 times higher than in the general population. Paediatric studies have suggested an even higher SMR for all children with epilepsy of 7–13.2;[4–6] however, in these studies the SMR for those children who have idiopathic epilepsy without any neurological or cognitive deficits is reported to be no higher than for their respective reference, non-epileptic populations.[4–6] In approximately 25% of cases death may be related directly to seizures (status epilepticus, accidental injury and sudden unexplained death [SUDEP]).[7] However, these data – and particularly SUDEP data – are primarily derived from adult populations.

There is very little information on the death rates of children with epilepsy, and in particular the risk of sudden unexpected death.[8–10] Death in a child with epilepsy may be due to:

1. **A complication of a seizure**
   aspiration
   suffocation
   injury (including burns)
   drowning
2. **Status epilepticus (convulsive)**
3. **A related underlying condition**
   tuberous sclerosis
   neurodegenerative disorder
   severe cerebral palsy

Sudden, unexpected death in epilepsy may be defined as; *'The sudden, unexpected, witnessed or unwitnessed, non-traumatic and non-drowning death in patients with epilepsy, with or without evidence for a seizure and excluding convulsive status epilepticus in which postmortem examination does not reveal a toxicological or anatomical cause for death'* (Nashef L. Sudden unexpected death in epilepsy: terminology and definitions. *Epilepsia* 1997; **38 (Suppl. 11):** S6–S8).

Data from the Office for National Statistics revealed the following deaths for paediatric epilepsy (excluding status epilepticus) in England and Wales in 2001 (asthma deaths are included for comparison):

	Epilepsy	Asthma
0–14 years	*36*	*23*
0–19 years	*64*	*36*
deaths/million population		
(0–14 yrs)	*37*	*11*

Deaths due to status epilepticus and status asthmaticus in the same period were as follows:

	Status epilepticus	Status asthmaticus
0–14 years	*12*	*3*
0–19 years	*14*	*3*

(Data from the National Statistics Office are considered to be reasonably accurate. As they are dependent on appropriate and accurate coding of disease and cause of death, any misdiagnosis may influence the data; this may be particularly relevant to epilepsy, where there are potential misdiagnosis rates of 25–30%.)

Certain characteristics are known to be associated with an increased risk of death:

- Epilepsy with onset in the first 12 months of life
- Epilepsy which is symptomatic in aetiology (e.g. cerebral malformation)
- Severe myoclonic epilepsies of infancy and early childhood
- Infantile spasms (related principally to the treatment of spasms – steroids and ACTH)
- Severe developmental delay already present at the onset of epilepsy

Sudden unexplained (or unexpected) death in epilepsy (SUDEP) is a phenomenon which has received much attention in the literature on adults, where it has been reported as being responsible for up to 15% of the mortality is epilepsy.[9] Most reports have focused on adult patients, although a small number of children have also been described. A retrospective, community-based paediatric study identified that, of 93 children with epilepsy who died over a five-year period, 11 (12%) died unexpectedly.[4] Children with secondary or symptomatic (rather than primary or 'idiopathic') epilepsy were at greater risk. No difference was noted in all-cause mortality rates between children with primary epilepsy and children without epilepsy. Mean age at death (for all 93 children) was 6.7 years; there were no age data for children dying suddenly and unexpectedly.

Two recent paediatric population studies confirm that although there is an increased risk of dying prematurely from epilepsy, most of these deaths occur in children/adolescents with severe neurological deficits. In the Dutch Study of Epilepsy in Childhood, 9 of 472 children who developed epilepsy between the ages of 1 month and 16 years died during the first five years of follow-up.[5] However, no deaths occurred in 328 children with idiopathic epilepsy, including patients with typical absence, juvenile myoclonic and benign rolandic epilepsy. The nine children who died all had symptomatic epilepsy and additional physical and/or learning difficulties. The study found no children died by drowning and no child died from SUDEP.[5]

In a Canadian study of 692 children in a single province (Nova Scotia) who developed epilepsy between 1977 and 1985, 26 had died by 1999, this rate of death being 5.3 and 8.8 times higher than those of the reference populations in the 1980s and 1990s respectively.[6] Twenty-one of the 26 deaths had occurred in children with severe neurological deficits. This meant that children with epilepsy and additional neurological problems were 22 times more likely to die than those without any neurological problem – an identical finding to the Dutch study. The

rate of SUDEP was also very low at 1.1/10 000 patient years.

It is possible that sudden unexplained death (in all ages) is under-estimated. Hypotheses to account for the phenomenon include a fatal cardiac arrhythmia (possibly representing an autonomic seizure), a severe, prolonged disturbance of brain-stem function by epileptic discharges or neurogenic pulmonary oedema (least likely). Episodes of bradycardia have been reported in a number of patients with complex partial seizures.

How does one counsel or inform parents of children with epilepsy, if at all, about sudden unexplained death? Some would inform all, others none, on the basis that the phenomenon is rare, affects only a small proportion (of all children with epilepsy) and is unpredictable and therefore unpreventable. Findings from a recent Nationally conducted clinical audit of epilepsy-related death have also suggested that the care patients (of all ages) received prior to death may, in some cases, have contributed to their premature death.[11]

Risk factors in *adults* include:[10]

- *Young age (18–30)*
- *Male sex*
- *Irregular use of antiepileptic medication*
- *Low serum levels of anticonvulsant drugs*
- *Generalized (tonic–clonic) convulsions*
- *Infrequent seizures*
- *Underlying structural brain abnormalities*
- *Sleep*

Although SUDEP may occur in children, it is likely to be rare. As yet, there is too little information on SUDEP in children to know which, if any, of the above risk factors apply and whether any new ones may be identified.

The Dutch and Canadian population studies, and to a lesser extent the National Sentinel Clinical Audit,[11] have provided some additional and important clinically useful information that should be of assistance in talking about this issue to families of children with epilepsy.[12]

Prevention of epilepsy

Perhaps somewhat surprisingly, there has been little research and little discussion within the literature about this potentially important aspect of epilepsy. In view of the fact that a significant proportion of epilepsy in childhood (up to 30–40%, possibly higher) has a genetic basis and given that for most of these patients genetic 'modification' will never be practicable or clinically justified (irrespective of the ethical dimension), it is unlikely that many of these epilepsies will ever be 'preventable'. For over a decade it has been claimed that with a greater understanding of the molecular (pathophysiological and genetic) basis of epilepsy, including the relatively newly discovered channelopathies, there would be novel and targeted treatments for the epilepsies, including possible prevention. Unfortunately and not unexpectedly, this has not – and is unlikely – to become a reality within even the next decade.

Obviously, where epilepsy is a common and disabling manifestation of a genetic and neurodegenerative disorder, such as the neuronal ceroid lipofuscinoses, genetic modification and/or therapy may be justifiable, although still not necessarily feasible.

Nevertheless there are many situations where the prevention of epilepsy or consequences of epilepsy will be both desirable and achievable; this is particularly applicable, but certainly not exclusive, to the developing world:

- Reduced incidence of high-risk, including teenage, pregnancies
- Improved monitoring and ante-natal care of women with high-risk pregnancies
- Improved perinatal care and prevention of any secondary brain damage – particularly in extremely premature and very low birth-weight infants
- Identification of any neuroprotective therapies that may reduce or prevent any secondary brain damage following an initial primary insult in early life
- Earlier recognition and appropriate treatment of meningitis, encephalitis and intracranial abscesses, particularly in infants and young children
- Improved uptake of childhood immunizations to reduce both the acute encephalopathies and the delayed complications associated with these illnesses (e.g. mumps and measles encephalitis and subacute sclerosing panencephalitis [SSPE])

- Improved road safety and traffic-exclusion measures to reduce the incidence of traumatic brain injury and post-traumatic epilepsy
- Improved resuscitation of children with acquired traumatic and non-traumatic brain injury and the prevention of secondary brain damage
- Correct identification and aggressive management of the relatively rare but important epileptic encephalopathies (e.g. West's syndrome, Landau–Kleffner syndrome, pyridoxine dependency) and non-convulsive status epilepticus, that if unrecognized may potentially cause irreversible cognitive impairment
- Avoidance of using inappropriate antiepileptic drugs, and specifically drugs that may exacerbate seizures
- Avoidance of the use of multiple antiepileptic drugs and in high doses that may have an adverse effect on concentration and short-term memory that, even if transient, may still irreversibly reduce educational potential (e.g. poor examination results)
- Early rather than late surgery for medically intractable epilepsy, particularly in mesial temporal lobe epilepsy where it may prevent irreversible psychosocial and cognitive (memory) impairment
- Improved pre-, intra-, and post-operative neurosurgical access (availability) and care for children requiring a surgical treatment for their epilepsy
- Identification of the child's (and the family's, including siblings') understanding and perceptions of epilepsy to prevent any additional psychopathology within the family
- Improved awareness, knowledge and understanding of epilepsy – what it is and what it is not – amongst all health-care and education professionals and the public to reduce, if not eliminate, the stigmatization of and not infrequent prejudice against all people with epilepsy

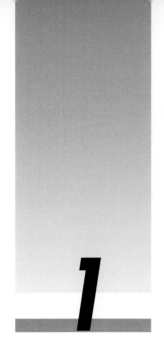

Diagnosis

The diagnosis of epilepsy should be considered at four
levels:

- *Recognition of epileptic seizures*
- *Classification of the seizure type or types (see page 17)*
- *Identification of the epilepsy syndrome (see page 20)*
- *Determination of aetiology (see page 49)*

Recognizing epileptic seizures is obviously essential in
making a diagnosis of epilepsy; in most cases it is
possible to classify the seizure type. For children and
adolescents it is important to attempt to then identify a
specific syndrome. Finally, a cause of the epilepsy
should always be considered and, when appropriate,
sought.

Recognition of epileptic seizures

The recognition and diagnosis of epileptic seizures is
almost entirely dependent on the history. The
examination will often be normal, and the results of any
investigations can only be interpreted with reference to
the history. A detailed description is required of events
occurring before, during and after a suspected epileptic
seizure. The accurate account of any eyewitness is
essential and will be the only history available when

young children present with seizures. Video-recordings of suspected seizures are a particularly useful aid to diagnosis and should be actively encouraged whenever there is any continuing doubt or confusion from the history. If the diagnosis is uncertain from the history then it is appropriate to await further episodes, since a delay in making a diagnosis of epilepsy is unlikely to be harmful. Undertaking investigations in the hope of confirming the diagnosis following an equivocal history increases the probability of making a false diagnosis of epilepsy, with potentially serious consequences for the child and family.[13]

Differential diagnosis of epilepsy

There are many conditions in childhood and adolescence that may be mistaken for epilepsy.[14,15] Disorders that are most commonly misdiagnosed as epilepsy include pallid syncopal attacks (also called reflex anoxic seizures), blue breath-holding attacks and night terrors in young children, and vasovagal syncope and migraine in older children. Failure to obtain an adequate history and interpreting stiffening, jerking, urinary incontinence or an abnormal EEG as invariably indicating an epileptic seizure are the most common reasons for making a false diagnosis of epilepsy.[16]

Episodes without altered consciousness

Jitteriness is a common condition, and startle disease or hyperekplexia is a rare disorder affecting the newborn. Both these conditions may be mistaken for seizures and are described further on page 73.

In benign myoclonus of early infancy, brief bursts of myoclonic-like spasms commence during the first year of life, occurring mainly while the infant is awake, but occasionally also during sleep. These spasms may resemble those seen in West's syndrome except that the EEG is normal, developmental progress remains unaffected and the spasms resolve by 2–3 years of age, if not earlier.

Abnormal head movements accompany vomiting in infants with benign paroxysmal torticollis. Writhing neck movements, sometimes associated with opisthotonic posturing, are occasionally seen in children with hiatus herniae in association with gastro-oesophageal reflux (Sandifer's syndrome).[17]

Fully conscious infants or children may have brief (seconds) shuddering or shivering episodes during which the arms and shoulders stiffen and tremor vigorously;[18] these can occur many times a day but are completely benign. The episodes may be triggered by excitement or stress; it is possible that they may represent a type of early tic or mannerism. Young children with benign paroxysmal vertigo suffer episodes of vertigo during which they appear suddenly frightened, pale and poorly co-ordinated; there is no confusion or drowsiness following the episodes. The diagnosis is often unclear until the child is old enough to describe the vertigo.

Children frequently display a variety of repetitive, ritualistic movements, including body rocking, motor tics or elaborate writhing and dystonic limb movements, even whilst fully conscious. The child may also appear flushed, distant or 'vacant', especially if there is a masturbatory element to these repetitive movements.

Paroxysmal choreoathetosis is a rare condition in which unilateral or bilateral dystonic movements, induced either by movement (i.e. kinesigenic), stress or coffee, occur up to several times a day, lasting from a few minutes to several hours. A dystonic drug reaction due to an anti-emetic or major tranquillizers should also be considered.

Older children and adolescents may experience anxiety states. These include panic attacks that could be mistaken for partial seizures with accompanying psychic or autonomic symptoms. Furthermore, any carpopedal spasm resulting from prolonged hyperventilation could be misinterpreted as an epileptic motor phenomenon, specifically a tonic seizure.

The episodes that may occur without exhibiting altered consciousness are summarized in *Table 3*.

Episodes of altered consciousness

Infants may occasionally present with recurrent episodes of loss of consciousness due to intermittent strangulation or suffocation by a parent. These episodes never occur in the absence of the abusing parent. A less alarming variant of this Munchausen's syndrome by proxy, or Meadow's syndrome, exists where a parent, usually the mother (and often with a medical or nursing background), fabricates a history of epilepsy in her child.[19,20]

Table 3
Episodes without altered consciousness and their typical age at presentation.

Episodes without altered consciousness	Typical age at presentation
Jitteriness	Infancy
Benign myoclonus of early infancy	Infancy
Benign paroxysmal torticollis	Infancy
Gastro-oesophageal reflux	Infancy and childhood
Shuddering attacks	Infancy and childhood
Startle disease (hyperekplexia)	Infancy and childhood
Benign paroxysmal vertigo	Childhood
Tics and ritualistic movements	Childhood
Paroxysmal choreoathetosis	Childhood and adolescence
Anxiety states	Adolescence
Drug-induced dystonias	Any

A contentedly daydreaming child may not always respond promptly to being called or touched. Although absence seizures and daydreaming both occur when a child is bored, absences will also interrupt activities, including speaking or eating.

Staring is usually a non-epileptic phenomenon in children and can usually be distinguished by a careful clinical history.[21] Staring spells or day-dreaming are commonly misdiagnosed by teaching staff as absence seizures. Non-epileptic staring spells seen in the classroom are often seen in children who may be tired, bored or occasionally in children with learning difficulties.

Blue breath-holding attacks are common in early childhood. An angry, frustrated child cries vigorously, then holds his breath, turns blue, becomes limp, loses consciousness for several seconds and may briefly stiffen or jerk; rarely these clonic movements may persist for many minutes.[22] Pallid syncopal attacks, also known as reflex anoxic seizures, are equally dramatic.[23] Following a sudden fright or injury the child cries briefly – following which there is a self-limiting bradycardia or asystole, leading to a brief loss of consciousness accompanied by pallor, during which, as in blue breath-holding episodes, stiffening or a few clonic jerks may be observed. Blue breath-holding attacks and reflex anoxic seizures may occur in the same child. The child usually returns to normal after a few minutes and only rarely falls asleep.

Vasovagal syncope is most commonly misdiagnosed as epilepsy in older children and adolescents. Simple faints are invariably provoked (by, for example, menstruation, prolonged standing, intercurrent illness), during which the child becomes cold, clammy and pale, and then slumps or falls stiffly to the ground, remaining unconscious for up to several minutes. Characteristically, just before losing consciousness, subjects experiencing a vasovagal syncope perceive a sheet of blackness sweeping across their field of vision. If generalized stiffening or clonic jerks and perhaps urinary incontinence occur, these features may suggest an epileptic seizure; however, brief tonic or clonic movements may occur in 75–80% and urinary incontinence in 5–10% of people during faints, blue breath-holding attacks and pallid syncopal attacks as a result of transient cerebral ischaemia and anoxia/hypoxia, and are *not* epileptic. For all these forms of neurally mediated syncope reassurance is appropriate and specific treatment is rarely required.[22,23]

Older children and adolescents may exhibit pseudo-epileptic or non-epileptic seizures.[24] These are included under episodes with altered consciousness since although consciousness is not actually altered, to an observer a subject exhibiting a pseudo-epileptic seizure usually appears to be unconscious. Pseudo-epileptic seizures are normally less stereotyped and of briefer duration than epileptic seizures, and sometimes appear quite bizarre, with pelvic thrusting, flailing and rolling movements.

Occasionally the seizures may be of considerably longer duration and, if mimicking a tonic–clonic seizure, the movements may wax and wane before suddenly ceasing; this is in contrast to a genuine tonic–clonic convulsion, which, as the clonic phase resolves, is characterized by movements which become less frequent but more marked before gradually coming to a stop. During a genuine tonic–clonic seizure the tongue is frequently bitten and the eyes are typically open; in contrast, during a pseudo-epileptic tonic–clonic seizure the tongue is rarely bitten and the eyes are shut – and there is voluntary resistance if an observer tries to open the eyes. Post-ictal drowsiness or confusion is rare. The absence of either ictal activity in the EEG or post-ictal slowing of the EEG is strongly suggestive of a pseudo-epileptic seizure. Prolactin levels are increased following an epileptic, but not after a non-epileptic tonic–clonic, convulsion; prolactin levels usually show no increase after complex partial, absence or myoclonic seizures.

Provided non-epileptic pseudoseizures are recognized then outcome in children and adolescents is encouraging with appropriate psychology and psychiatry support, and is much better than that reported in adults.[24–26] Outcome is less favourable for males (who form the minority of those affected by pseudoseizures), for those not identified until late adolescence and for those who also have true epileptic seizures in addition to non-epileptic

pseudoseizures.[26] Non-epileptic pseudoseizures need to be managed sensitively because in some cases this problem is a manifestation of dysfunctional family relationships and in other cases the sufferers may have been subjected to violence, physical/sexual abuse or neglect, although sometimes pseudo-epileptic seizures are part of attention seeking or avoidance behaviour.[25,26]

Visual disturbances, altered body image, ataxia and reduced level of consciousness may be experienced during the aura of classical migraine or basilar artery migraine, and may be misinterpreted as 'epileptic'. The visual aura in migraine usually lasts for many minutes and is characterized by geometric shapes and patterns that are white, silver or gold. In contrast, the visual 'aura' of a simple or complex partial seizure tends to be of considerably shorter duration and the images are often definite objects (including people) or circles and multi-coloured (red, green, blue, yellow, purple).

The irresistible urge to sleep (which may occur anywhere, at any time, and may last for only a few minutes) that is characteristic of narcolepsy may occasionally be mistaken for a complex partial seizure. Cataplexy, or the sudden loss of muscle tone, which is another feature of narcolepsy, may also be misdiagnosed as an epileptic seizure (atonic or myoclonic seizure). Cataplexy is always precipitated – by laughter, excitement or a sudden startle. Altered consciousness, abnormal behaviour and perceptual disturbances feature in certain epileptic seizures but may also occur either as part of the delirium that sometimes accompanies febrile illnesses or in association with substance abuse. Apparent epileptic seizures that recur only in association with intercurrent illnesses and fasting should prompt investigation of a possible underlying metabolic disorder.

Cardiac arrhythmias[27] such as the prolonged QT interval or Wolf–Parkinson–White syndromes should be suspected if convulsions or episodes of loss of consciousness occur during, or shortly after, exercise or at times of a sudden shock or fright. Cerebral hypoxia due to cardiac dysrhythmias should also be considered as a cause of atonic or tonic seizures, as this seizure type rarely occurs in isolation in neurologically normal children.

The episodes that result in an apparent altered consciousness are summarized in *Table 4*.

Episodes related to sleep

In benign sleep myoclonus of infancy, a young infant may have intermittent myoclonic jerks during sleep which start from a few days of age; these jerk may last many minutes, but they never involve the face and do not wake the child. The EEG is normal, and the jerks cease by 3–6 months of age, although occasionally they may persist to 8 or 9 months, if not longer.

Hypnagogic and hypnopompic phenomena

Table 4
Episodes of altered consciousness and their typical age at presentation.

Episodes with altered consciousness	Typical age at presentation
Meadow's syndrome	Infancy and childhood
Daydreaming	Childhood
Ritualistic movements	Childhood
Blue breath-holding attacks	Childhood
Pallid syncopal attacks	Childhood
Vasovagal syncope	Childhood and adolescence
Pseudo-epileptic seizures	Childhood and adolescence
Migraine	Childhood and adolescence
Narcolepsy	Childhood and adolescence
Substance abuse	Adolescence
Delirium	Any
Metabolic disorders	Any
Cardiac arrhythmias	Any

may occur at any age, and comprise myoclonus, auditory hallucinations and even brief visual hallucinations on falling asleep or on awakening.

Children can be very restless during normal sleep and some children indulge in elaborate, ritualistic movements while settling in bed. Occasionally, young children may rhythmically jerk their heads while falling asleep or indulge in head banging which appears dramatic but does not cause injury; these movements should not be confused with either myoclonic or clonic seizures.

Night terrors are not uncommon in young children. After one or two hours' sleep the child suddenly sits up, screams, and appears terrified, but is not actually awake, and will resume sleeping after many minutes with no subsequent recollection of the event. However, it may be very difficult to differentiate night terrors from frontal lobe complex partial seizures. One helpful, though not invariable differentiating, feature is that frontal lobe seizures are usually multiple (many occurring in a single night), in contrast to night terrors, which usually occur only once per night. In addition, the duration of a frontal lobe complex partial seizure is usually considerably shorter than that of a night terror. Sleepwalking, another type of parasomnia, is also common, but more frequently occurs in older children; rarely there may be some associated semi-purposeful behaviour which may resemble the automatisms that are a feature of certain complex partial seizures.

The episodes related to sleep are summarized in *Table 5*.

Table 5
Episodes related to sleep and typical age at presentation.

Episodes related to sleep	Typical age at presentation
Benign sleep myoclonus of infancy	Infancy
Head bobbing or banging	Infancy and childhood
Night terrors	Childhood
Ritualistic movements	Childhood
Hypnagogic movements	Childhood and adolescence
Sleepwalking	Childhood and adolescence

Classification of epilepsies

2

Epileptic seizures

Seizures are classified into either generalized or partial seizures *(Table 6)*.[28] The whole brain (or at least the whole of the cerebral cortex) is involved in generalized seizures, whereas partial seizures only affect part of the brain. Partial seizures are also called focal or localized seizures. Partial seizures are further classified as 'simple', in which consciousness is retained, or 'complex', in which consciousness is impaired or lost. Simple partial seizures with sensory, autonomic or psychic symptoms may easily be overlooked in younger children unable to describe such symptoms. Partial seizures may become secondarily generalized, resulting in a tonic–clonic convulsion. The symptoms of a simple partial seizure prior to secondary generalization constitute the epileptic aura.

A recent diagnostic scheme proposal has been submitted to the International League Against Epilepsy. The scheme encompasses five divisions, or axes: seizure description, seizure type, epilepsy syndrome, aetiology and associated impairment. This proposed scheme is under debate but the classifications of seizures and of syndromes from the scheme are considered in this chapter because these include seizures and syndromes that have been recognized since the current international classifications were formally accepted.

The seizure classification in the proposed diagnostic scheme prefers the term 'focal' to 'partial' or 'localized' or 'local'. It is proposed that the terms 'simple' and 'complex' should be dropped in favour of describing, in individual patients, whether consciousness is fully preserved, impaired or lost during focal seizures.[29] This diagnostic scheme is a 'work-in-progress' and has not replaced the seizure classification shown in *Table 6*. However, this proposed scheme contains several additional seizure types not included in the older classification. Inhibitory motor seizures and gelastic seizures appear in the focal group, eyelid myoclonia and spasms are added under generalized

Table 6
Classification of seizures.

Partial seizures (seizures beginning locally)

Simple (consciousness not impaired)
   With motor symptoms
   With somatosensory or special sensory symptoms
   With autonomic symptoms
   With psychic symptoms
Complex (with impairment of consciousness)
   Beginning as simple partial seizures, progressing to complex seizures
   Impairment of consciousness at onset
      1. Impairment of consciousness only
      2. With automatism
Partial seizures becoming secondarily generalized

Generalized seizures

Absence seizures
   Typical (petit mal)
   Atypical
Myoclonic seizures
Clonic seizures
Tonic seizures
Tonic–clonic seizures
Atonic seizures

(From Commission on Classification and Terminology of the International League Against Epilepsy. Proposal for revised clinical and electroencephalographic classification of epileptic seizures. Epilepsia 1981; 22: 489–501.)[28]

seizures, and negative myoclonic and reflex seizures are listed in both groups.

Consciousness is severely impaired or lost during a generalized seizure, although this may only be transient if the seizure is very brief. Therefore, for a person to be aware of symptoms during a seizure, the seizure is likely to have been partial or, if the seizure appeared to have been generalized, then there was probably a partial onset.

In a tonic seizure there is a sustained, forceful, rigid contraction of the affected part of the body (usually the whole body). In contrast, in a clonic seizure affected muscles contract and relax rhythmically, usually with the contraction phase being more rapid than the relaxation phase. The amplitude of the clonic contraction tends to increase whilst the rhythm slows towards the end of the seizure. In a tonic–clonic seizure the sustained contraction, typically lasting 10–20 seconds, is followed by rhythmic contractions, often for several minutes.

During absence seizures, there is a brief loss of consciousness causing the affected person to become unresponsive and to stare but there is not usually any loss of posture. Automatisms are common, occurring in at least 50% of children and typically involve the lips (lip-smacking, chewing, swallowing) or hands (fidgeting or washing movements). A slight flickering of the eyelids sometimes occurs during absence seizures but in eyelid myoclonia there is more vigorous rapid blinking as the eyes deviate upwards. Although absences may occur in those experiencing eyelid myoclonia, such absences are independent of the episodes of eyelid myoclonia. On recovery from an absence, the child or teenager is often – but not always – aware that 'something happened', but they cannot recall any more details.

Myoclonic seizures comprise extremely rapid, very brief muscular contractions that occur either singly or are repeated only a few times. Myoclonic seizures may occur in prolonged bouts, but there are brief periods of muscular relaxation between the seizures, in contrast to clonic seizures, in which rhythmic contractions persist throughout the period of seizure activity. A sudden, brief reduction in muscle tone, causing a loss of posture, occurs in atonic seizures. Atonic seizures are often associated with myoclonic seizures. In negative myoclonic seizures, inhibitory activity within the primary motor cortex is abnormally enhanced and cessation of muscle activity either occurs in isolation (pure negative myoclonus) or during the cortical slow wave that follows the spike activity of a preceding myoclonic movement (complex negative myoclonus). Negative myoclonus is rare.

Spasms are seizures in which there are sudden, widespread, muscular contractions (typical examples occurring in infantile spasms). Although spasms were formerly considered to be massive myoclonic seizures, they are now regarded as a separate seizure type. The new, proposed classification includes 'epileptic spasms' as a specific seizure type; 'infantile' spasms occur in the first 13–14 months of life and 'epileptic' spasms occur in later childhood. Appropriately, the proposed new classification recognizes that both types of spasms may be either focal or generalized in origin. The differentiation of a myoclonic seizure, epileptic spasm or tonic seizure may be difficult on clinical grounds alone. However, the EEG correlate and the muscle activity recorded on electromyography (EMG) are characteristically different for each seizure type:

Seizure type	Duration of seizure	EEG correlate
Myoclonic	<1 second	Polyspike discharge
Spasm	1–2 seconds	Slow-wave discharge or flattening on the EEG
Tonic	>5 seconds	Fast spiking

Reflex seizures, either generalized or focal, are manifest by abnormal cortical discharges causing muscular activity (usually tonic, myoclonic or clonic in nature) and occur in response to a variety of sensory stimuli.

Numbness or tingling of part of the body is a common symptom of somatosensory seizures. Motor seizures (often clonic) may affect only part of the body as a result of focal, abnormal cerebral cortical activity. Inhibitory motor seizures are rare and arise from excessive, focal cortical inhibitory activity producing temporary muscular weakness, usually affecting one or more limbs. In psychic seizures there may be feelings of fear, rage or elation, although such seizures could also be manifest by visual, auditory or olfactory hallucinations. Psychic seizures arise from the temporal lobe and may be accompanied by semi-purposeful – even automatic – activities during which the affected person is vague and unresponsive (automatisms). The combination of a psychic seizure and an automatism is known as a psychomotor seizure.

Autonomic phenomena occur during various types of seizure and include pupillary changes, alterations in pulse rate and blood pressure, vomiting, salivation and skin colour changes. In critically ill patients who require muscle paralysis and ventilation, sudden unexplained changes in autonomic function may provide the only clinical indication of epileptic seizure activity unless some form of cerebral electrical recording is utilized. However, there should be a high threshold for diagnosing epileptic seizures on clinical grounds alone in critically ill patients, particularly those requiring ventilatory support and sedation (on the intensive care unit). In this situation advice from a paediatric neurologist is important. Continuous cerebral electrical activity monitoring may be useful (e.g. continuous cerebral function analysis monitoring or CFAM).[30] Finally, gelastic seizures consist of outbursts of laughter, but laughter that is inappropriate and also 'hollow' or even unpleasant.

Epilepsies and epileptic syndromes

The epileptic seizure type is one criterion used to define epileptic syndromes. Epileptic syndromes are determined by:

- Seizure type(s)
- Age of onset
- EEG findings (interictal and ictal)
- Associated features, such as neurological findings, family history

Epileptic syndromes are important in the management of epilepsy in terms of:

- Predicting prognosis
- Selecting treatment
- Defining the likelihood of identifying an underlying aetiology

The classification of epilepsies and epileptic syndromes is divided, according to the topographic origin of seizures, into those where the origin of the seizure is localization-related (i.e. partial or focal) and those that are generalized (*Table 7*).[31] A further subdivision is made

aetiologically into symptomatic, in which the cause of the epilepsy is known, cryptogenic, in which there is a likely, but unidentified, cause, and idiopathic, in which there is no underlying cause apart from perhaps a genetic predisposition. International classifications of epilepsy are unlikely to be entirely satisfactory, and reservations have been expressed particularly with respect to seizure classification in infants.[32] However, these classifications are of practical value in permitting an international dialogue on the diagnosis and treatment of epilepsy and in facilitating collaborative research. To remain clinically valid, these classifications will clearly need to evolve in the light of experience and as a result of new research. Regular classification revisions are to be anticipated in the near future, particularly in view of the current rapid expansion in the understanding of genetic aspects and basis of epilepsy.

Table 7
ILAE classification of epilepsy.

1. Localization-related (focal, local, partial) epilepsies and syndromes
1.1 Idiopathic (with age-related onset) – benign childhood epilepsy with centro-temporal spikes – childhood epilepsy with occipital paroxysms – primary reading epilepsy 1.2 Symptomatic – chronic progressive epilepsia partialis continua of childhood (Kojewnikow's syndrome) – syndromes characterized by seizures with specific modes of presentation 1.3 Cryptogenic (presumed symptomatic but aetiology unknown)

Continued

Table 7 Continued

2.	**Generalized epilepsies and syndromes**

2.1   Idiopathic (with age-related onset, listed in order or age)
- benign neonatal familial convulsions
- benign neonatal convulsions
- benign myoclonic epilepsy in infancy
- childhood absence epilepsy
- juvenile absence epilepsy
- epilepsy with grand mal (generalized tonic–clonic seizures) on awakening
- other generalized idiopathic epilepsies not defined above
- epilepsies with seizures precipitated by specific modes of activation (reflex and reading epilepsies)

2.2   Cryptogenic or symptomatic (in order of age)
- West's syndrome
- Lennox–Gastaut syndrome
- epilepsy with myoclonic–astatic seizures
- epilepsy with myoclonic absences

2.3   Symptomatic

    2.3.1   Non-specific aetiology
- early myoclonic encephalopathy
- early infantile epileptic encephalopathy with suppression burst
- other symptomatic generalized epilepsies not defined above

    2.3.2   Specific syndromes/aetiologies
- cerebral malformations
- inborn errors of metabolism, including pyridoxine dependency and disorders frequently presenting as progressive myoclonic epilepsy

3.   **Epilepsies and syndromes undetermined, whether focal or generalized**

3.1   With both generalized and focal seizures
- neonatal seizures
- severe myoclonic epilepsy in infancy
- epilepsy with continuous spike-waves during slow-wave sleep
- acquired epileptic aphasia (Landau–Kleffner syndrome)
- other undetermined epilepsies not defined above

3.2   Without unequivocal generalized or focal features

4.   **Special syndromes**

4.1   Situation-related seizures
- febrile convulsions
- isolated seizures or isolated status epilepticus
- seizures occurring only when there is an acute metabolic or toxic event due to factors such as alcohol, drugs, eclampsia, non-ketotic hyperglycinaemia
- reflex epilepsy

*(From Commission on Classification and Terminology of the International League Against Epilepsy. Proposal for classification of epilepsies and epileptic syndromes. Epilepsia 1989; **30**: 389–99.)*[31]

The recently proposed diagnostic scheme for epilepsy includes an epilepsy syndrome classification *(Table 8)*.[29] For syndromes, as for seizures, it is suggested that the terms 'partial' or 'localization-related' should be dropped in favour of the term 'focal'. It is also proposed that the phrase 'probably symptomatic' should be used in preference to the former term 'cryptogenic' and that epilepsy syndromes that are symptomatic or probably symptomatic should be grouped together. The generalized syndrome category in the proposed scheme only contains idiopathic syndromes and a new category entitled epileptic encephalopathies is included in which epileptiform abnormalities appear to contribute to progressive cerebral dysfunction. These epileptic encephalopathies are not further divided into generalized, focal, idiopathic or symptomatic, perhaps because of continuing uncertainty regarding firstly the aetiology of some of these syndromes and secondly whether they represent focal or generalized epilepsies.

Table 8
A proposed scheme for epilepsy syndromes (2001).

FOCAL (PARTIAL, LOCALIZATION-RELATED) EPILEPSIES
Idiopathic
- Benign infantile seizures (non-familial)
- Benign childhood epilepsy with centro-temporal spikes
- Early-onset benign childhood occipital epilepsy (Panayiotopoulous type)
- Late-onset childhood occipital epilepsy (Gastaut type)

Familial (autosomal dominant)
- Benign familial neonatal seizures
- Benign familial infantile seizures
- Autosomal dominant nocturnal frontal lobe epilepsy
- Familial temporal lobe epilepsy

Symptomatic (or probably symptomatic)
- Limbic epilepsies
- Mesial temporal lobe epilepsy with hippocampal sclerosis
- Mesial temporal lobe epilepsy defined by specific aetiologies
- Other types defined by location and aetiology
- Neocortical epilepsies
- Kojewnikow's syndrome (Rasmussen's encephalitis)
- Hemiconvulsion–hemiplegia syndrome
- Other types defined by location and aetiology

GENERALIZED EPILEPSIES
Idiopathic
- Benign myoclonic epilepsy in infancy
- Epilepsy with myoclonic astatic seizures
- Childhood absence epilepsy

Continued

Table 8 *Continued*

- Epilepsy with myoclonic absences
- Juvenile absence epilepsy
- Juvenile myoclonic epilepsy
- Epilepsy with generalized tonic–clonic seizures only
- Generalized epilepsies with febrile seizures plus

REFLEX EPILEPSIES
- Idiopathic photosensitive occipital lobe epilepsy
- Other visual sensitive epilepsies
- Primary reading epilepsy
- Startle epilepsy

EPILEPTIC ENCEPHALOPATHIES
- Early myoclonic encephalopathy
- Ohtahara syndrome
- West's syndrome
- Dravet syndrome (severe myoclonic epilepsy in infancy)
- Lennox–Gastaut syndrome
- Landau–Kleffner syndrome
- Epilepsy with continuous spike-waves during slow-wave sleep

PROGESSIVE MYOCLONIC EPILEPSIES

SEIZURES NOT NECESSARILY REQUIRING A DIAGNOSIS OF EPILEPSY
- Benign neonatal seizures (non-familial)
- Febrile seizures
- Reflex seizues
- Alcohol-withdrawal seizures
- Drug- or chemically induced seizures
- Immediate and early post-traumatic seizures
- Single, isolated clusters or rarely repeated seizures

*(Derived from Engel J. A proposed diagnostic scheme for people with epileptic seizures and with epilepsy: report of the ILEA task force on classification and terminology. Epilepsia 2001; **42**: 796–803.[29])*

The new proposed diagnostic scheme for epilepsy syndromes *(Table 8)*, is a work-in-progress and has not replaced the current, well-established classification of epilepsy syndromes *(Table 7)*. However, this new proposed diagnostic scheme is shown because it includes additional epilepsy syndromes that have been identified in recent years and may, in future, lead to modification of the current epilepsy syndrome classification.

Epileptic syndromes of childhood and adolescence[33]

The main epileptic syndromes of childhood and adolescence are discussed in this section. In 30–40% of children it may not always be possible to identify an epileptic syndrome, particularly at the time of the child's initial presentation, although inter-rater agreement is good and most syndromes can be identified at the time of initial diagnosis.[34,35]

Benign idiopathic neonatal convulsions ('fifth day fits')

Prevalence	Rare (<1% of all childhood epilepsy)
Age of onset	Day 1–7, most around day 5
Seizure type(s)	Partial clonic or subtle (e.g. apnoea)
EEG – Interictal	Asynchronous rolandic theta rhythm
– Ictal	Rhythmic spikes or slow waves
Aetiology	Idiopathic
Treatment	Phenobarbitone, phenytoin, benzodiazepines; none
Prognosis	Excellent; seizures do not usually recur when medication is withdrawn
Other features	Autosomal dominant inheritance (chromosome 20), possibly related to a disorder of potassium channels

Benign familial neonatal convulsions

Prevalence	Rare (<1% of all childhood epilepsy)
Age of onset	Day 2–3, but occasionally up to 3 months
Seizure type(s)	Generalized clonic, occasionally tonic
EEG	The ictal recording often begins with generalized flattening followed by either generalized spike and wave or some focal discharges. Although considered a generalized epilepsy syndrome, asymmetrical EEG features in this syndrome and in benign idiopathic neonatal convulsions possibly results from immaturity of the corpus callosum
Aetiology	Idiopathic
Treatment	Phenobarbitone, carbamazepine, valproate
Prognosis	Good; seizures cease by 6 months but 11% develop other epilepsies (that are usually readily controlled)
Other features	Autosomal dominant inheritance (chromosome 20)

Early myoclonic encephalopathy (neonatal myoclonic encephalopathy)

Prevalence	Rare (<1% of all childhood epilepsy)
Age of onset	Neonatal period
Seizure type(s)	Fragmentary (segmental, erratic) myoclonic, generalized myoclonic and partial motor, evolving after several months into infantile spasms
EEG – Interictal and Ictal	Bursts of spikes, sharp waves and slow waves alternating with virtually silent periods (burst-suppression) evolving into atypical hypsarrhythmia **(Figure 2)**
Aetiology	Metabolic disorders, including non-ketotic hyperglycinaemia, rarely found
Treatment	Corticosteroids, benzodiazepines, valproate, vigabatrin but usually no effective therapy
Prognosis	Poor; all infants are neurologically abnormal and 50% die within a year

In the syndrome of early infantile epileptic encephalopathy (Ohtahara's syndrome) that begins in the first months of life, brief tonic seizures are the main seizure type, the EEG shows burst-suppression, but with longer bursts than in early myoclonic encephalopathy, and brain malformations are common

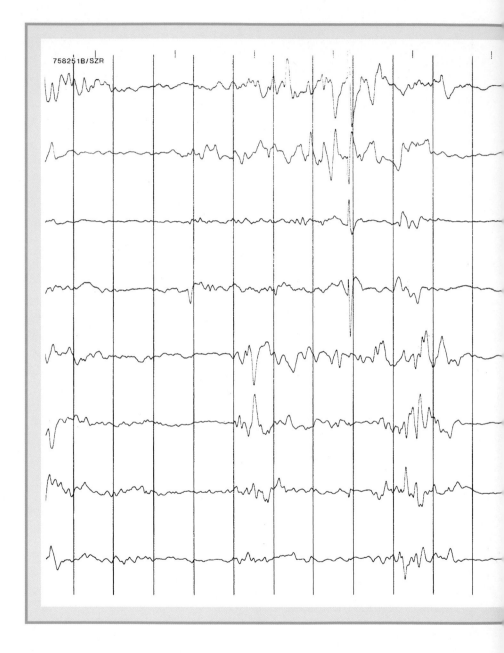

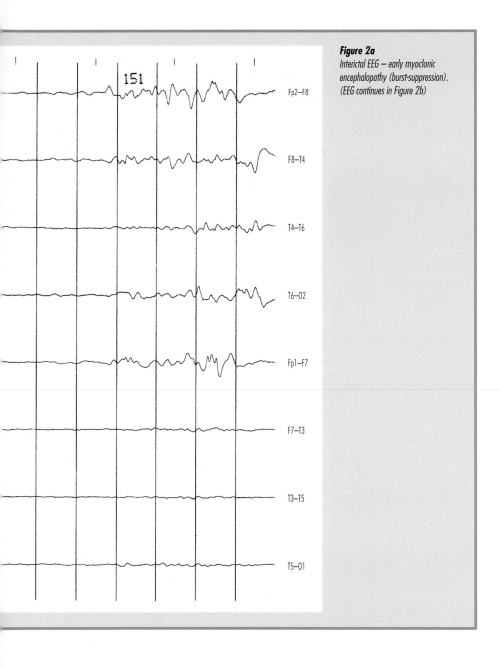

Figure 2a
*Interictal EEG – early myoclonic
encephalopathy (burst-suppression).
(EEG continues in Figure 2b)*

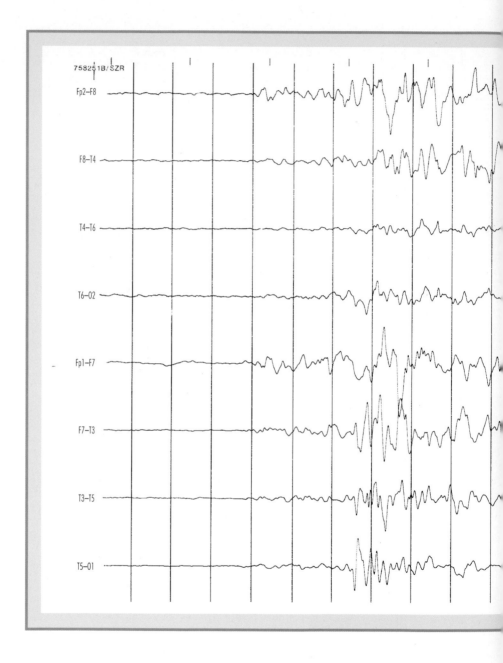

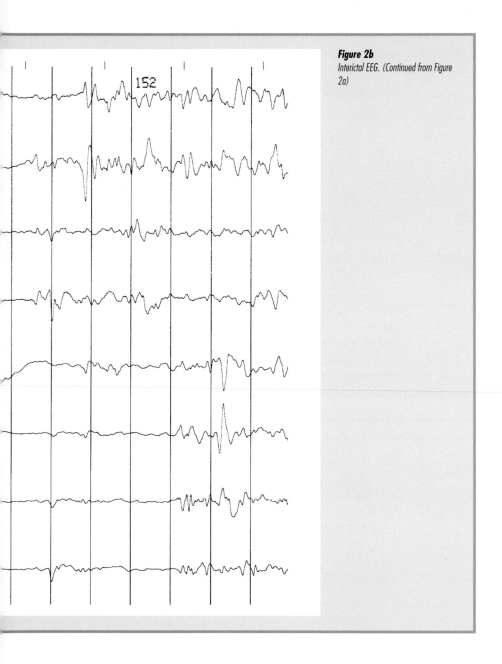

Figure 2b
Interictal EEG. (Continued from Figure 2a)

Benign infantile focal seizures (familial and non-familial)

Prevalence	Rare (< 1% of all childhood epilepsy)
Age of onset	First 2 years of life
Seizure type(s)	Initial motor arrest with staring followed by a convulsion (focal clonic or tonic–clonic or secondarily generalized), often occurring in clusters
EEG – Interictal	Normal
– Ictal	Focal discharges (sometimes becoming secondarily generalized)
Aetiology	Sporadic or, in some cases, familial
Treatment	Valproate, carbamazepine, phenobarbitone
Prognosis	Good response to treatment with generally good developmental outcome. In some familial cases paroxysmal choreoathetosis rarely develops during childhood or adolescence either at rest or induced by exertion or anxiety

Malignant migrating partial seizures in infancy

Prevalence	Very rare (<< 1% of all childhood epilepsy).
Age of onset	First 6 months of life
Seizure type(s)	Focal clonic, or tonic–clonic, becoming very frequent with autonomic features (apnoea, flushing, cyanosis)
EEG – Interictal	Diffusely slow
– Ictal	Rhythmic theta, initially focal becoming generalized with frontal predominance
Aetiology	Unknown
Treatment	Various, including steroids and benzodiazepines; stiripentol; no drugs are usually effective
Prognosis	Very poor developmental outcome; some show no developmental progress and some die in the first few years of life

Pyridoxine (vitamin B6) dependency [36,37]

Prevalence	Unknown
Age of onset	In utero – 18 months (peak, first week of life)
Seizure type(s)	Multifocal or generalized (myoclonic, tonic or clonic). Frequent. (Infantile spasms have also been described)
EEG – Interictal	Markedly abnormal; hypsarrhythmic-like, burst-suppression or multifocal discharges
Treatment	Pyridoxine dosage in newborn – 50–100 mg bd; dose in older children 3–30 mg/kg per day. Clinical response to intravenous pyridoxine is usually immediate, as is normalization of the EEG, although the latter may be delayed for days or weeks. In suspicious or equivocal cases a trial of oral pyridoxine should be given for at least 4 weeks. Any infant under the age of 18 months with intractable seizures should receive a 4-week trial of pyridoxine
Prognosis	Poor if diagnosis made late; even with early diagnosis and treatment, children may show marked psychomotor delay
Other features	Pyridoxine acts as a co-factor for the enzyme glutamic acid decarboxylase in the synthesis of the inhibitor neurotransmitter GABA. Autosomal recessive inheritance. The condition may also be seen in infants with structural lesions of the brain – again emphasizing the importance of using a pyridoxine trial 'diagnostically' in any infant with a cerebral abnormality and seizures that are refractory to conventional anti-epileptic drugs

West's syndrome (infantile spasms and hypsarrhythmia)[38,39]

Prevalence	Uncommon (1–5% of all childhood epilepsy)
Age of onset	3–13/14 (peak 5–9) months
Seizure type(s)	Brief tonic or clonic spasms, typically in clusters recurring many times daily. Spasms are commonly flexor–extensor (neck and arms flex, legs extend), but may be flexor (jack-knife; salaam attacks) or extensor. Occasionally seizures consist only of 'head nods'
EEG – Interictal	Chaotic; large-amplitude slow waves with spikes and sharp waves varying in site and size (hypsarrhythmia). At onset, hypsarrhythmia may only be seen when drowsy or during light sleep. Atypical hypsarrhythmia is common in symptomatic cases (variable mixture of asymmetry, focal elements, burst-suppression and preservation of basal rhythm) **(Figure 3)**
– Ictal	High-amplitude slow wave followed by diffuse fast rhythms or flattening (electrodecrementation) of trace
Aetiology	70–80% symptomatic (perinatal hypoxic–ischaemic encephalopathy, malformations including tuberous sclerosis, pre- and post-natal infections, metabolic disorders, e.g. phenylketonuria). 20–30% cryptogenic/idiopathic, although subtle cerebral dysplasias may not be apparent on neuro imaging until around 2 years of age
Treatment	Vigabatrin, steroids (prednisolone, tetracosactrin [ACTH]), valproate, nitrazepam, lamotrigine, topiramate, pyridoxine, immunoglobulins
Prognosis	Generally poor and generally worse if symptomatic. 70% have severe developmental delay, 5–10% will have normal developmental progress, 50–60% develop other epilepsies (especially Lennox–Gastaut syndrome)
Other features	Male/female = 1.5:1.0. The triad of spasms, hypsarrhythmia and arrested psychomotor development typifies this syndrome, although the spasms and hypsarrhythmia are the two key defining criteria

Benign myoclonic epilepsy of infancy

Prevalence	Rare (<1% of all childhood epilepsy)
Age of onset	4 months–3 years
Seizure type(s)	Brief generalized myoclonic, often as falling asleep
EEG – Interictal	Generalized spikes or polyspikes
Aetiology	Idiopathic
Treatment	Valproate, (benzodiazepines, lamotrigine)
Prognosis	Good, although generalized tonic–clonic seizures sometimes occur in adolescence and delayed treatment in infancy may be associated with psychomotor problems
Other features	Male/female = 2:1

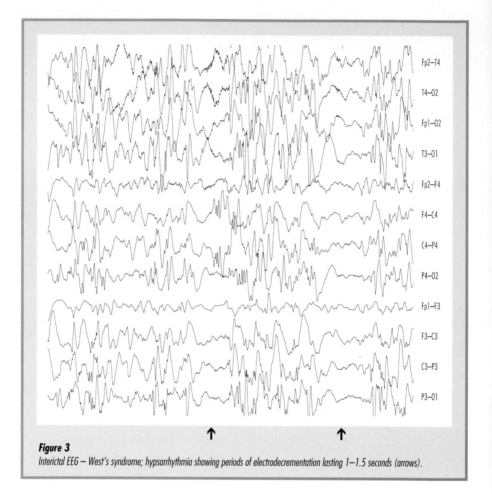

Figure 3
Interictal EEG – West's syndrome; hypsarrhythmia showing periods of electrodecrementation lasting 1–1.5 seconds (arrows).

Severe myoclonic epilepsy in infancy (Dravet syndrome)

Prevalence	Rare (<1% of all childhood epilepsy)
Age of onset	3–8 months
Seizure type(s)	Febrile seizures (frequently prolonged) often occur in the first year of life, followed at age 15–24 months by frequent generalized or segmental myoclonic seizures. 40–50% also have atypical absences and/or partial motor seizures, possibly with secondary generalization
EEG – Interictal	Generalized spikes, variable focal abnormalities, photosensitivity
– Ictal	Fast spikes and polyspikes with myoclonic seizures
Aetiology	Possibly idiopathic; possible genetic basis
Treatment	Valproate, benzodiazepines, topiramate, ethosuximide, stiripentol
Prognosis	Poor. Intractable seizures, developmental delay (particularly in speech and language), progressive pseudo-ataxia (because of frequent seizures and markedly abnormal EEG, even without obvious clinical seizures)
Other features	Male/female = 2:1.

Lennox–Gastaut syndrome

Prevalence	Uncommon (1–5% of all childhood epilepsy), but the most common intractable childhood epilepsy. Over-diagnosed.
Age of onset	1–8 (peak 3–5) years
Seizure type(s)	Tonic, atypical absences (begin and end gradually), atonic and myoclonic. Massive myoclonic and atonic seizures both cause sudden falls ('drops'). Episodes of both convulsive and, more frequently, non-convulsive status epilepticus (complex partial and atypical absence) are common, recurrent and often difficult to treat
EEG – Interictal	Awake = slow (1.0–1.5 Hz) spike and slow wave **(Figure 4)**; asleep = fast (10 Hz) spike bursts
– Ictal	Tonic – diffuse fast bursts; atypical absences – diffuse 1.0–1.5 Hz spike and slow waves; myoclonic or atonic – diffuse spikes or polyspikes and slow waves
Aetiology	Cryptogenic or symptomatic
Treatment	Valproate, lamotrigine, topiramate, carbamazepine (for tonic seizures), benzodiazepines, steroids, ketogenic diet, immunoglobulins, corpus callosotomy
Prognosis	Poor; seizures gradually reduce, but developmental and later cognitive difficulties persist and are usually severe or even profound. Patients become fully dependent on carers
Other features	At least 20% have preceding West's syndrome. A variety of other intractable epilepsies with mixed seizure types but without the above EEG features are sometimes incorrectly included under this syndrome

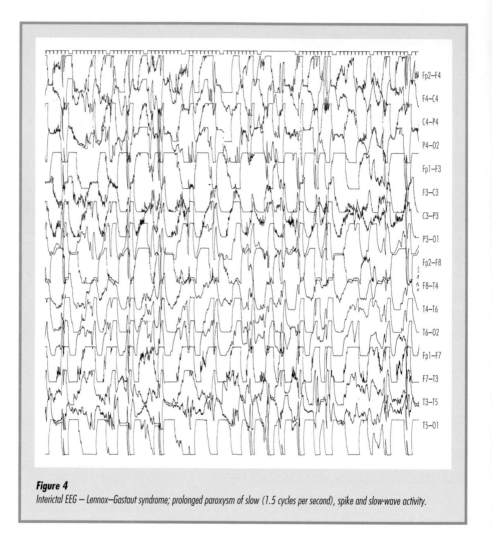

Figure 4
Interictal EEG – Lennox–Gastaut syndrome; prolonged paroxysm of slow (1.5 cycles per second), spike and slow-wave activity.

Myoclonic–astatic epilepsy

Prevalence	Uncommon (1–5% of all childhood epilepsy)
Age of onset	1.5–5 years
Seizure type(s)	Generalized myoclonic and myoclonic–astatic causing falls. Tonic–clonic, absence and tonic seizures also often occur
EEG – Interictal	2–3 Hz bursts of (poly)spike and wave
– Ictal	(Poly)spike and wave, either isolated or in 2–3 Hz runs, followed by a brief silent period
Aetiology	Probably genetic (15–40% – family history of epilepsy)
Treatment	Valproate, ethosuximide, benzodiazepines, lamotrigine, topiramate (and possibly levetiracetam)
Prognosis	Variable, sometimes reasonable outcome with seizure control and no major learning difficulties

This syndrome differs from the Lennox–Gastaut syndrome in that myoclonic seizures are the predominant seizure type, the outcome is better and the syndrome may have a genetic basis. The original description by Doose included some cases of benign and severe myoclonic epilepsy of infancy

Progressive myoclonic epilepsies

There are a number of rare myoclonic epilepsies occurring during childhood in which generalized or fragmentary myoclonic seizures, and often other seizure types, are associated with neurological deterioration including cerebellar impairment and cognitive dysfunction. Most are degenerative (progressive):

Continued

1. Disorders in which clinical presentation is _typically_ progressive myoclonic epilepsy

Lafora body disease
Ramsay–Hunt syndrome – also called
Unverricht–Lundborg syndrome (Baltic myoclonus, or dyssynergia cerebellaris myoclonica)
Sialidosis Type 1 (cherry red spot myoclonus syndrome)
Sialidosis Type 2
Mucolipidosis Type 1
Juvenile neuropathic Gaucher's disease (Type 3)
Juvenile neuroaxonal dystrophy

2. Disorders in which clinical presentation is _occasionally_ progressive myoclonic epilepsy:

Ceroid lipofuscinoses
– early and late infantile forms
– early and late juvenile forms
Myoclonic epilepsy with ragged-red fibres ('MERRF')
Huntington's disease
Wilson's disease
Hallervorden–Spatz disease

3. Disorders in which clinical presentation is _atypical_ progressive myoclonic epilepsy:

Non-ketotic hyperglycinaemia
Infantile hexosaminidase deficiency
– Tay–Sachs disease
– Sandhoff's disease
Biopterin deficiency
Sulphite oxidase deficiency

Specific treatments are available for only a few of the underlying metabolic disorders. Myoclonic seizures may respond to valproate plus benzodiazepines, ethosuximide, topiramate, piracetam, levetiracetam and possibly baclofen or chloral hydrate but can be aggravated by carbamazepine, gabapentin, vigabatrin and sometimes phenytoin. Piracetam may be particularly helpful in many of these syndromes – including in the ceroid lipofuscinoses

Hemiconvulsions, Hemiplegia, Epilepsy (HHE) syndrome

Prevalence	Very rare (<< 1% of all childhood epilepsy)
Age of onset	0–4 years
Seizure type(s)	Initial prolonged hemiclonic (one side of body) followed by hemiparesis of variable duration (sometimes with permanent hemiplegia). Complex partial seizures (often of temporal lobe origin) develop several years later
EEG – Ictal	Hemiclonic seizures: 2–3 Hz bilateral slow waves with variable, faster discharges over contralateral hemisphere. Subsequent complex partial seizures: focal discharges (e.g. as in mesial temporal lobe epilepsy syndrome)
Aetiology	Fever provokes initial hemiclonic convulsions. Pathogenesis of subsequent unilateral (sometimes bilateral) cerebral atrophy may be similar to, but much more severe than, mesial temporal sclerosis
Treatment	Prolonged hemiconvulsions – treat as for status epilepticus. Subsequent complex partial seizures – treat as in the mesial temporal lobe epilepsy syndrome
Prognosis	Earlier reports gave poor outcome for seizure control, motor function and development but the syndrome is becoming increasingly rare with better prognosis (possibly due to improved treatment of prolonged febrile seizures and episodes of status epilepticus)

Early-onset benign childhood occipital epilepsy (Panayiotopoulos type)

Prevalence	Common (approximately 5% [possibly 10%] of all childhood epilepsy)
Age of onset	1–13 (peak 3–6) years
Seizure type(s)	Prolonged autonomic features, often vomiting, with eye deviation and decreased consciousness. Frequently begins during sleep and lasts from minutes to several hours. Often followed by a unilateral clonic convulsion or a generalized tonic–clonic (occasionally tonic) convulsion. Full recovery occurs after a post-ictal sleep although sometimes there is a post-ictal headache
EEG – Ictal	Multi-focal (occipital in 2/3 of cases), sharp and slow-wave discharges
Aetiology	Idiopathic
Treatment	Rectal diazepam for prolonged seizures. Carbamazepine for recurrent seizures (but as only a single seizure occurs in 1/3 of cases, treatment may not always be necessary)
Prognosis	Excellent; a minority with recurrent seizures will resolve within a couple of years. 5–10% may develop benign rolandic epilepsy.

Panayiotopoulos syndrome is a broader concept than occipital epilepsy, representing an early-onset benign childhood seizure susceptibility syndrome (not always associated with occipital discharges) that may form a continuum with febrile seizures in younger children and benign rolandic epilepsy in older children

Late-onset childhood occipital epilepsy (Gastaut type)

Prevalence	Rare (< 1% of all childhood epilepsy)
Age of onset	3–16 (peak 8) years
Seizure type(s)	Frequent (often daily), brief (seconds to 2 minutes), visual hallucinations – typically multicoloured circles but sometimes more complex figures. Eye deviation, eyelid flickering and blindness for several minutes may occur. Occasionally terminates with a hemiclonic or generalized tonic–clonic convulsion. Post-ictal headache occurs in 50%, and 10% of these also vomit
EEG – Interictal	Occipital spikes (possibly only during sleep)
– Ictal	Fast, occipital spikes
Aetiology	Idiopathic
Treatment	Carbamazepine
Prognosis	Fair – 60% remit within a few years

The frequency, nature and brevity of the visual hallucinations should help to distinguish this syndrome from the visual aura of migraine

Typical absence epilepsy of childhood

Prevalence	Common (5–12% of all childhood epilepsy)
Age of onset	3–12 (peak 6–7) years
Seizure type(s)	Absences with prompt onset and cessation of impaired consciousness lasting 5–15 seconds and recurring 10–100+ times daily. Often accompanied by eyelid flutter and automatisms, including lip-smacking, chewing and hand-fidgeting
EEG – Interictal	Paroxysmal single or brief generalized spike-wave discharges
– Ictal	Generalized, symmetrical, 3–3.5 Hz spike-wave discharges **(Figure 5)**
Aetiology	Idiopathic (genetic in most)
Treatment	Valproate, ethosuximide, lamotrigine (singly or in combination)
Prognosis	Variable. Seizures remit in 65–70% but in 40% tonic–clonic seizures develop in adolescence; myoclonic seizures are very rare; up to 30% of children may show subtle cognitive impairment
Other features	Male/female = 1.5. Hyperventilation (undertaken for 4 minutes) frequently induces absences and is a very useful test in the clinic. This syndrome is also known as 'petit mal', but this term should now be avoided

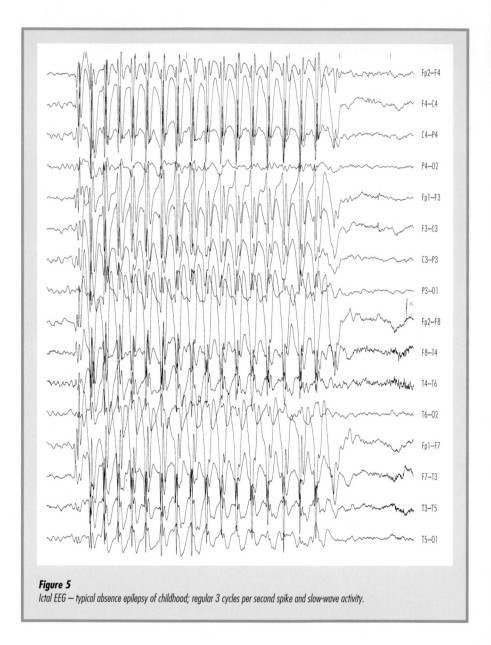

Figure 5
Ictal EEG – typical absence epilepsy of childhood; regular 3 cycles per second spike and slow-wave activity.

Epilepsy with myoclonic absences *develops usually in boys aged 1–12 years, with absences associated with generalized myoclonic seizures. The EEG is similar to that in typical absence epilepsy, but treatment with valproate and ethosuximide (usually combined) is less effective; lamotrigine or clobazam/clonazepam may be effective. Developmental delay is common*

Juvenile absence epilepsy *is similar to typical absence epilepsy of childhood, but with a later onset of 9–17 (peak 9–12) years. Absences occur less frequently but last longer and during them the child/teenager may still be able to perform certain, and even relatively complicated, tasks although they are not usually able to speak. This may lead to an initial (false) diagnosis of complex partial seizures – and inappropriate treatment (carbamazepine). The EEG shows spike and slow-wave activity but at a faster rate (3.5–4.5 Hz); the EEG may also show asymmetric activity – which may also contribute to an initial, false diagnosis of partial epilepsy. Most also have tonic–clonic seizures, especially on awakening, and some have myoclonic seizures. Treatment is as for childhood-onset absences; prognosis is not as favourable*

Benign partial epilepsy with centro-temporal (rolandic) spikes

Prevalence	*The most common partial epilepsy of childhood: 10–15% (?20%) of all childhood epilepsy*
Age of onset	*3–13 (peak 7–9) years*
Seizure type(s)	*Partial sensorimotor. Sensory aura (unilateral paraesthesiae) is followed by a unilateral tonic and/or clonic seizure involving the tongue, lips, cheek, larynx, pharynx and occasionally the arm. 70–75% of seizures occur during sleep or on awakening. Consciousness is preserved if awake but secondary generalization is common if asleep*
EEG – Interictal	*Unilateral or bilateral centro-temporal spikes* **(Figure 6)**
– Ictal	*Discharge remains localized, or becomes secondarily generalized*
Aetiology	*Idiopathic; may be genetic*
Treatment	*Carbamazepine or oxcarbazepine; lamotrigine or topiramate may be alternatives; none (if seizures few and infrequent)*
Prognosis	*Excellent; seizures cease spontaneously (usually by puberty), but initially may be frequent*

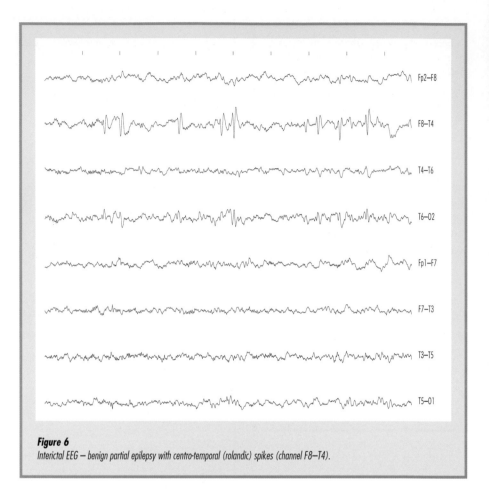

Figure 6
Interictal EEG – benign partial epilepsy with centro-temporal (rolandic) spikes (channel F8–T4).

Benign partial epilepsy with occipital paroxysms is not rare; patients aged from 1 to 17 years experience seizures with positive visual symptoms (amaurosis, illusions or hallucinations which are multicoloured), sometimes accompanied by eye deviation and vomiting, followed by hemiclonic seizures or automatisms and often a post-ictal headache. Spike-waves are seen uni- or bilaterally in the occipital region on eye closure, and may spread to the central region during a seizure. A family history of epilepsy and/or migraine is common

Landau–Kleffner syndrome (acquired epileptic aphasia)[33,40]

Prevalence	Rare; probably under-diagnosed
Age of onset	2–10 (peak 5–7) years
Seizure type(s)	Infrequent generalized tonic–clonic or partial motor. Usually preceded (sometimes followed) by a severe receptive and expressive language disorder leading to aphasia, but with normal hearing and audiometry

EEG – Interictal	Awake = multifocal spike and spike-wave discharges in temporal or parieto-occipital regions. Sleep = bursts of slow spike-waves during slow-wave sleep often prolonged and at times almost continuous
Aetiology	Unknown
Treatment	Corticosteroids (initial preferred treatment for a short period); clobazam, valproate, lamotrigine, surgery (subpial transection)
Prognosis	Good for seizure control, poor for language recovery. Seizures usually cease spontaneously by age 15–16 years
Other features	Male/female = 2:1. Psychomotor and behavioural difficulties are very common, and are more of a problem than the seizures. 20% have aphasia and EEG abnormality without seizures

Spike-wave discharges during slow-wave sleep are commonly seen in the Landau–Kleffner syndrome. In the rare syndrome of **epilepsy with continuous spike-waves during slow-wave sleep (electrical status epilepticus during slow sleep [ESESS]),** this EEG pattern occupies at least 85% of slow-wave sleep in children aged from 1–12 years who may experience a variety of seizure types. Developmental (including language) regression is very common

Chronic progressive epilepsia partialis continua of childhood (Kojewnikow's or Rasmussen's syndrome)

Prevalence	Rare (<1% of all childhood epilepsy)
Age of onset	Within first 10 years
Seizure type(s)	Frequent, continuous, partial motor
EEG – Interictal and Ictal	Spikes and spike-waves predominantly unilateral in fronto-temporal region with widespread slow activity
Aetiology	A relatively localized subacute encephalitis (Rasmussen's encephalitis) of uncertain aetiology. Mitochondrial encephalomyopathies. Cryptogenic
Treatment	Drug treatment, except possibly steroids or intravenous immunoglobulins, usually ineffective. Hemispherectomy may be the only effective treatment and should be considered early
Prognosis	Poor; progressive hemiplegia, dysphasia and intellectual disability

Generalized epilepsy with febrile seizures plus[41]

Prevalence	May be common (> 5% of all childhood epilepsy), but unclear at present
Age of onset	Febrile seizures within the first 5 years, other seizures later in childhood
Seizure type(s)	Typical febrile seizures in early childhood. Various seizures appear later in childhood (tonic–clonic, absence, myoclonic, atonic, partial motor, or continuing brief, febrile generalized seizures)
EEG – Interictal and Ictal	Normal or generalized epileptiform discharges
Aetiology	Probably autosomal dominant. Various mutations of sodium channels
Treatment	Standard antiepileptic medication depending on seizure type(s)
Prognosis	Fair; development usually satisfactory, seizure control variable

The mesial temporal lobe epilepsy syndrome[42]

Prevalence	Uncommon (1–5% of all childhood epilepsy), but a common cause of intractable seizures
Age of onset	Initial febrile (or afebrile) seizures at 0–4 years of age, then epilepsy during childhood or adolescence
Seizure type(s)	Complex partial seizures, usually lasting 1–2 minutes, sometimes with secondary generalization. Aura common (e.g. epigastric sensation, emotional disturbance) followed by oral, hand, verbal automatisms and semi-purposeful behaviour
EEG – Interictal	Unilateral (sometimes bilateral) anterior–mid-temporal spikes (best seen with depth electrodes)
– Ictal	Rhythmic 5–9 Hz sharp waves from temporal lobe (may be missed by scalp electrodes), sometimes with secondary generalization
Aetiology	Mesial temporal sclerosis (hippocampal sclerosis), sometimes bilateral but asymmetrical, in 70% of adults requiring resection (higher proportion of dysplasias and low-grade gliomas in childhood). It is uncertain whether the mesial temporal sclerosis is the cause or consequence of recurrent febrile seizures
Treatment	Carbamazepine, topiramate, lamotrigine, oxcarbazepine. As add-on (especially with carbamazepine), levetiracetam, clobazam, acetazolamide. Surgery – anterior temporal lobectomy or selective amygdalohippocampectomy
Prognosis	Approximately 60% reasonable control on medication. If amenable to surgery, seizure control is usually excellent (75–80% achieve a 'cure' and antiepileptic medication can be withdrawn)
Other features	Behavioural and memory disturbances are common and often progressive

Juvenile myoclonic epilepsy (Janz syndrome)[43]

Prevalence	5–10% of all epilepsy; the most common epilepsy syndrome in adolescence; often not correctly recognized
Age of onset	Peak 12–16; range 8–26 years
Seizure type(s)	Bilateral, single or multiple myoclonic seizures predominantly in the arms. Generalized tonic–clonic seizures also occur in 90%, with juvenile-type absences in 10–30%. Seizures related to sleep deprivation, occurring shortly after awakening, or when drowsy
EEG – Interictal	Normal, or brief discharges resembling ictal trace **(Figure 7)**. Photosensitivity common (40–70% of cases) **(Figure 8)**
– Ictal	Rapid (>3 Hz), irregular, generalized spike and polyspike wave discharge
Aetiology	Idiopathic (genetic)
Treatment	Valproate, lamotrigine, acetazolamide, clobazam, topiramate and possibly levetiracetam; carbamazepine and phenytoin exacerbate myoclonic and absence seizures and should be avoided
Prognosis	Good; excellent response to valproate but seizures usually (60–70%) recur if therapy withdrawn
Other features	Family history of epilepsy is common. One gene associated with this syndrome may lie on chromosome 6; another possibly on chromosome 15; others likely

Epilepsy with grand mal (generalized tonic–clonic seizures) on awakening

Prevalence	Uncommon (1–5% of all childhood epilepsy)
Age of onset	6–20 (peak 11–15) years
Seizure type(s)	Generalized tonic–clonic soon after awakening or when relaxing. Additional seizures (myoclonic, absence) are relatively uncommon
EEG – Interictal	Occasional generalized spike-wave discharges with some excess of background slow rhythm
– Ictal	Generalized spike-wave discharges
Aetiology	Idiopathic (may have a genetic basis, similar to juvenile myoclonic epilepsy)
Treatment	Valproate, carbamazepine, lamotrigine, topiramate, gabapentin
Prognosis	Good. Seizures respond well to therapy but relapses are common (50–70% of people), if medication is withdrawn

Isolated partial seizures of adolescence

Prevalence	Uncommon (1–5% of all childhood epilepsy), but accounts for about 25% of unprovoked partial seizures in adolescence
Age of onset	10–19 (peak 13–15) years
Seizure type(s)	Simple and/or complex partial (with motor and/or sensory features)
EEG – Interictal	Normal
Aetiology	Idiopathic
Treatment	None or carbamazepine
Prognosis	Good; seizures may be very occasional
Other features	Male/female = 2:1

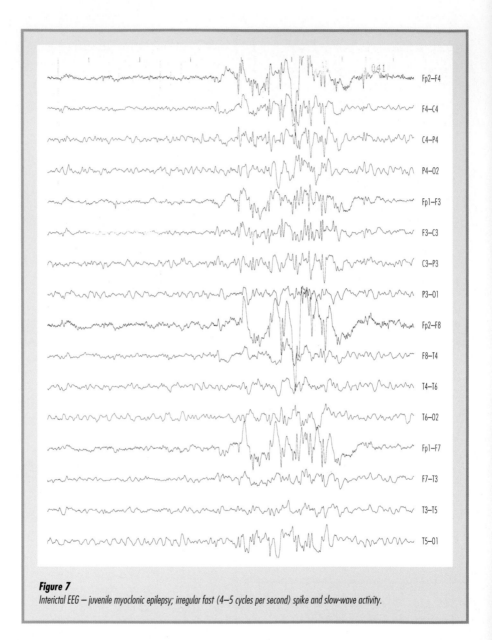

Figure 7
Interictal EEG — juvenile myoclonic epilepsy; irregular fast (4–5 cycles per second) spike and slow-wave activity.

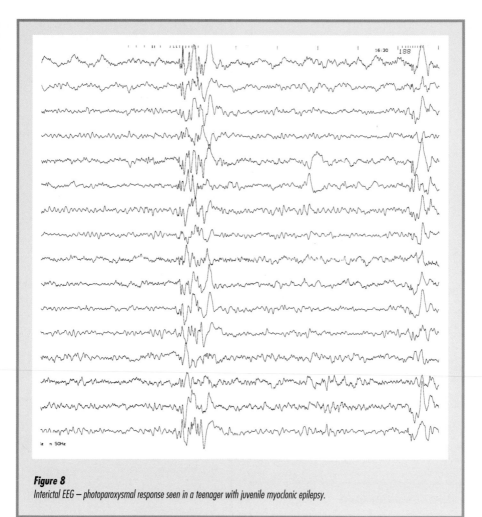

Figure 8
Interictal EEG – photoparoxysmal response seen in a teenager with juvenile myoclonic epilepsy.

Autosomal dominant nocturnal frontal lobe epilepsy[44,45]

Prevalence	Uncommon (1–5% of all childhood epilepsy)
Age of onset	0–50+ (85% < 25) years
Seizure type(s)	Brief (< 1 minute), stereotyped, tonic or dystonic with rapidly changing limb and trunk movements. Consciousness may be preserved
EEG – Interictal	Normal or anterior focal discharges
– Ictal	Rapid frontal sharp waves or spikes (but may be normal with standard scalp EEG)
Aetiology	Various nicotinic acetylcholine receptor mutations on chromosome 20
Treatment	Carbamazepine; lamotrigine and topiramate may also be effective.
Prognosis	Fair; seizures remit over several decades
Other features	Sleep deprivation and stress are provoking factors. Behavioural problems are common until seizures are well controlled

Familial temporal lobe epilepsy

Prevalence	Rare (< 1% of all childhood epilepsy)
Age of onset	1–60 (peak 15–19) years
Seizure type(s)	Simple and/or complex. Mesial form – psychic (especially déjà vu) and autonomic. Lateral form – auditory. Secondarily generalized tonic–clonic seizures also common in mesial form
EEG – Interictal	Normal or slow wave/spike and sharp wave over temporal lobes
Aetiology	Autosomal dominant

Treatment	Carbamazepine; lamotrigine and topiramate may also be effective
Prognosis	Seizures infrequent but 20% resistant to medication
Other features	MRI of temporal lobes is normal

Reflex epilepsies[33, 46–48]

There are a number of epilepsies that are triggered or induced by specific stimuli or situations, some of which may have a clear psychological component.

The reflex epilepsies are divided into a simple group induced by sensory (e.g. visual) stimuli or movements and a complex group induced by mental and emotional processes (e.g. reading).

- Photosensitive epilepsy (flicker- or flash-induced and pattern-induced)
- Reading epilepsy
- Startle epilepsy
- Musicogenic epilepsy
- Eating-induced epilepsy
- Immersion (hot or cold water)-induced epilepsy
- Mathematic or calculation-induced epilepsy

Photosensitive epilepsy is the most common and most relevant, in terms of its age and onset and management implications. Photosensitivity includes induction by flickering light of the right intensity and frequency or by specific visual patterns, and will produce characteristic paroxysms on the EEG which may or may not be accompanied by a photoconvulsive clinical response – in which the individual usually will have either a myoclonic or a tonic–clonic seizure.

One demographic study in Great Britain identified an annual incidence of cases with a newly presenting seizure and unequivocal photosensitivity of 1.1/100 000 (5.7/100 000 in the age group from 7 to 19 years). This means that photosensitivity is found in 2% of patients of all ages presenting with seizures and 10% of patients presenting with seizures in the age range 7–19 years.[49,50]

Photosensitivity rarely occurs in isolation; it is far more commonly seen in patients with idiopathic generalized epilepsies, usually with an age of onset from 10 to 18 years of age (particularly in juvenile myoclonic epilepsy, when it is seen in at least 40% and possibly as high as 80%[51] of individuals). Far less commonly, photosensitivity may be seen in children aged 2–6 years; in this age group it is relatively more common in children with the cryptogenic or symptomatic rather than the idiopathic generalized epilepsies (e.g. severe myoclonic epilepsy of infancy, myoclonic–astatic epilepsy and a number of the progressive myoclonic epilepsy syndromes). When occurring in the idiopathic generalized epilepsies it is far more common in girls, and the phenomenon usually resolves by the early–mid twenties. The most sensitive flicker rate is 14–20/sec, but rates as high as 25 and 50/sec (as found in television sets in the UK, but not in the USA, where the rate is 60/sec) may also induce seizures in photosensitive individuals.[49,52] Simple measures may reduce the risk of a photically induced seizure:

- Sitting at least 3 metres from a TV screen (or 1 metre from a computer screen if playing a video game)

- Using a remote control to change channels

- Watching TV or playing a video game with a bright light on in the room

- Covering one eye (with a hand, not just closing the eye) if approaching a TV set; this is because the visual stimulus causing photosensitivity has to be binocular

- Not playing a video game when excessively tired (tiredness and relative sleep deprivation lower the threshold for a photosensitive seizure). (The length of time played on a video game does not significantly influence the risk of having a photically induced seizure)

Sodium valproate is effective in suppressing both photo-paroxysmal responses (spike and slow waves) on the EEG and photically induced clinical seizures. No other antiepileptic drug is recognized (as yet) to be as effective, although lamotrigine and the benzodiazepines may also be beneficial.

The complex group of reflex epilepsies are rare, but of these the most common is reading epilepsy. This begins in adolescence whilst reading, is more common in males (approximately 2:1), and comprises simple partial, tonic and myoclonic seizures involving muscles used in speech. If reading continues then a secondarily generalized tonic–clonic convulsion may follow. Treatment involves stopping reading when simple partial seizures occur, or using valproate or clonazepam. Seizures are usually well controlled but complete remission is rare.

Aetiology of epilepsy

3

Epilepsy may be associated with almost any cerebral pathology and other cerebral dysgeneses *(Figure 9)*.[53–55] Although no specific cause will be found in 70–75% of children, an aetiology may be demonstrable from the clinical information and examination findings alone.

Malformations[56,57]

There is a high risk of epilepsy developing in children with neuronal migration disorders and other cerebral dysgeneses. Magnetic resonance imaging (MRI) is far superior to computed tomographic (CT) scanning in the detection of neuronal migration disorders. Various seizure types are associated with neuronal migration disorders, but partial seizures (sometimes with secondary generalization) and myoclonic seizures predominate. Neuronal migration abnormalities are generally fairly diffuse, but may be more prominent in a particular area of the brain, and in such cases if the EEG indicates this area to be the focus of seizures then epilepsy surgery could be considered. Many children with neuronal migration disorders have significant learning difficulties and epilepsy that is difficult to control, but this is not invariable (even when the abnormality on an MRI scan is fairly extensive); specifically, familial periventricular nodular heterotopia may present at any age with partial seizures that are relatively easy to control.

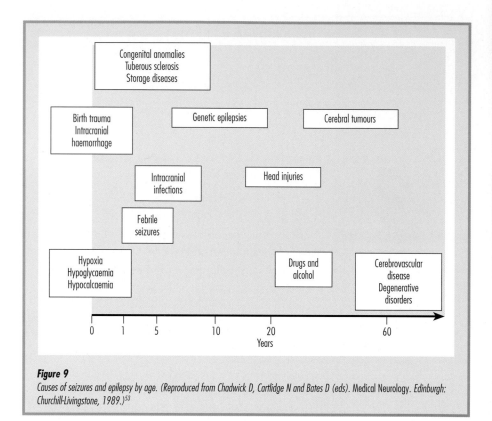

Figure 9
Causes of seizures and epilepsy by age. (Reproduced from Chadwick D, Cartlidge N and Bates D (eds). Medical Neurology. Edinburgh: Churchill-Livingstone, 1989.)[53]

Epilepsy is commonly associated with the cerebral malformations that occur in certain neurocutaneous syndromes, including the cortical tubers of tuberous sclerosis and the leptomeningeal angiomatosis of the Sturge–Weber syndrome. Approximately 60% of children with tuberous sclerosis have epilepsy, but this rises to almost 100% if there are associated severe learning difficulties. Epilepsy occurs in 60–90% of children with Sturge–Weber syndrome. Epilepsy is also relatively common in neurofibromatosis type1.

Miscellaneous syndromes

There are several hundred chromosomal abnormalities in which seizures feature, but there are only a few chromosomal disorders that are highly associated with epilepsy.[58] Up to 6–8% of children with Down's syndrome and 20–40% of people with the Fragile X syndrome develop epilepsy, including infantile spasms. The risk of epilepsy is also increased in other, less common, syndromes. In Rett's syndrome, affected girls show neurodevelopmental regression after initial normal early development, and 80%

develop seizures. Up to 80–90% of children with Angelman's syndrome develop seizures.

Metabolic disorders[59,60]

There are numerous metabolic disorders that can cause seizures, although most are rare. In previously healthy children and adolescents presenting with seizures, measurement of blood glucose and calcium are the only worthwhile routine metabolic investigations. Disorders of intermediate metabolism associated with seizures tend to present fairly dramatically in the neonatal period or in early infancy,[59,60] often at times of intercurrent illness or infection. These disorders can be broadly categorized by measuring the pH, glucose, lactate and ammonia in the blood and urinary ketones. Further elucidation and management of the suspected metabolic disorder requires liaison with a specialized clinical chemistry laboratory (see pages 74–77 for a further discussion of the investigation of seizures in neonates). Neurodegenerative disorders associated with epilepsy progress insidiously during infancy and childhood and many have an identifiable underlying metabolic defect. These disorders are usually suspected because of the associated neurological signs and developmental regression. Specific biochemical, histological or neurophysiological investigations are required to confirm the diagnosis.

Infections

The risk of epilepsy following meningitis or encephalitis is relatively small, but increases if seizures occur during the acute illness.[61,62] Epilepsy is up to five times more common in patients who convulse during their acute illness than in those who do not. β-Haemolytic streptococci and *Streptococcus pneumoniae* tend to be associated with acute seizures (and therefore later epilepsy); this may be related to age, as it is usually the younger child, including the neonate, who is infected with these particular bacteria. Ten per cent of children develop epilepsy after meningitis and 20% after encephalitis. Epilepsy develops in over 75% of patients requiring drainage of a cerebral abscess.

Pertussis vaccination, like other vaccinations, may produce a fever leading to febrile seizures in susceptible children, but the consensus is that pertussis vaccination does not cause brain injury and subsequent epilepsy (including infantile spasms).[63] Intractable seizures, including infantile spasms and the Lennox–Gastaut syndrome, may complicate congenital infections with toxoplasmosis, rubella, cytomegalovirus (CMV), herpes simplex, other viruses and syphilis.[64]

Head injury[65–68]

The majority of children who have a head injury do not experience a seizure. The overall risk of epilepsy developing after a head injury is approximately 5%, but it is slightly higher (between 7% and 9%) in children under 5 years of age.

Post-traumatic seizures can be classified into three types:

---

1. *Immediate – seizures occurring within the first 24 hours (usually within minutes) of the injury*
2. *Early – seizures occurring within the first week of the injury*
3. *Late – seizures occurring months to years following the injury*

The incidence of immediate or early seizures varies between 5% and 20% depending upon the severity of the injury. Early seizures are one of the major risk factors predisposing to late epilepsy. There are a number of factors which are associated with an increased risk of late epilepsy:

- *Immediate/early seizures*
- *Depressed skull fracture*
- *Intracranial haemorrhage/haematoma*
- *Focal cerebral damage (particularly if caused by a missile injury)*
- *Prolonged (i.e. >24 hours) post-traumatic amnesia*
- *A genetic predisposition towards epilepsy*

As expected, the greater the number of factors the greater is the chance of developing late epilepsy. Early post-traumatic seizures are correlated with an approximately 25% probability of late epilepsy. The rate increases to 40% if there has been an intracranial

haemorrhage and to 60–70% if most of the above factors have occurred. Prolonged post-traumatic amnesia and a genetic predisposition to epilepsy (as manifest by a family history of epilepsy) do not, in isolation, increase the risk of late epilepsy in the absence of all other risk factors. It is important to realize that all of the above risk factors are related to the primary brain injury and if there is any secondary brain damage then this will further increase the risk of both early and late seizures. This emphasizes the importance of the appropriate early management of both traumatic and non-traumatic brain injury in preventing any secondary cerebral damage.

Approximately 20% of children with late seizures will have their initial seizure in the first month following the head injury, while 50–60% of late seizures will occur within the first year. Almost 20% of children will start to develop late epilepsy as long as 4 years after the injury and the figure will have fallen to 10% or less by 6 years or longer.

The majority of early seizures are partial seizures and over half of all late seizures are generalized (more commonly secondary rather than primary generalized) seizures. Status epilepticus (convulsive) is uncommon – and is more likely to occur in the first few days after the injury and is seen more often in children than in adults, particularly if under 2 years of age and usually when the cause of the injury has been non-accidental and due to an hypoxic–

ischaemic cerebral insult. Non-convulsive status epilepticus is very uncommon in traumatic brain injury – and is more commonly seen in non-traumatic brain injury.

There remains some debate regarding the use of antiepileptic drugs to prevent the development of late epilepsy. Current evidence suggests that antiepileptic drugs do not reduce the risk and incidence of developing late epilepsy.[69–71] In one adult study of over 400 patients, 27% of patients treated with an anticonvulsant had developed late epilepsy at 2 years following the head injury, in contrast to only 21% of patients who had not received an anticonvulsant.[70] This same study did suggest, however, that using an anticonvulsant just for the first week after the head injury could reduce the risk of further seizures occurring in that week. It is the authors' current practice to prescribe phenytoin (following an initial intravenous 'loading' dose) if the child has had two or more seizures in the first few days following the head injury and to discontinue the drug after 2 or 4 weeks if the child has remained seizure-free. Should late epilepsy develop, the drug of choice will depend on the type of seizure and EEG findings but should not include phenytoin or phenobarbitone as drugs of first choice.

Hypoxic–ischaemic injury

Hypoxic–ischaemic cerebral injury resulting from cardiorespiratory arrest or drowning is a well-recognized, but rare,

antecedent of epilepsy in childhood. Hypoxic–ischaemic encephalopathy (HIE) in the perinatal period is a common cause of 'late' epilepsy, including infantile spasms (West's syndrome). West's syndrome arising because of a perinatal hypoxic–ischaemic encephalopathy is extremely difficult to treat. HIE is one of the 'worst' causes of infantile spasms. Hypoxic–ischaemic injury is likely to be the primary mechanism of damage in infants and young children subjected to non-accidental injury (often a shaking injury), through cerebral oedema and/or multiple shearing injuries throughout the brain.

Tumours

Cerebral tumours are a cause of seizures in less than 1–2% of children with epilepsy.[72] This reflects the usual infratentorial (posterior fossa or brain-stem) siting of paediatric tumours, particularly in children under 6 years of age. However, in children with brain tumours, 10–20% may present initially with one or more seizures;[73,74] these tumours are usually astrocytomas, primitive neuroepithelial tumours (PNETs) or dysembryoblastic neuroepithelial tumours (DNETs) and less commonly oligodendrogliomas or meningiomas. Many of these tumours are benign, and the epilepsy usually remits if the tumour is completely excised. EEG focal delta waves are a classical, but by no means universal, feature of cerebral tumours. MRI is more sensitive than CT scan at detecting small tumours and in identifying tumours such as PNETs and DNETs.

Haemorrhage

Spontaneous intracranial haemorrhage is rare in childhood, resulting from congenital vascular malformations or acquired disorders such as thrombocytopenia and neonatal vitamin K deficiency. Epilepsy follows a subarachnoid or intracranial haemorrhage in about 20% of subjects.

Dual pathology[75–77]

Improved structural and functional neuro-imaging techniques have demonstrated dual pathology, particularly in patients, including children, with intractable (usually partial) epilepsy. Most commonly this comprises hippocampal atrophy/mesial temporal sclerosis and another lesion. This 'other' lesion is usually an abnormality of neuronal migration (e.g. grey matter heterotopia or cortical dysplasia). Less commonly, vascular malformations, periventricular leucomalacia or low-grade tumours have been identified. The significance and relationship of dual pathologies is not clear; it is possible that they share a common pathogenesis (i.e. cause) with an onset during pre- or perinatal development. Alternatively, one lesion/abnormality may have caused the other; e.g. an area of cortical dysplasia may have been responsible for initiating early-onset and repeated seizures (with or without an associated 'febrile illness'), which consequently resulted in, or at least contributed to, the hippocampal atrophy/mesial temporal sclerosis. The identification of dual pathology is not just of academic interest; it has potential and important clinical implications when evaluating patients for surgical treatment for their partial epilepsy (see also Chapter 6 on Febrile seizures).

Febrile seizures

See Chapter 6.

Cerebral palsy[78,79]

Many of the previously discussed genetically determined and acquired disorders associated with epilepsy may also cause cerebral palsy. However, in up to 20% of children with cerebral palsy there are no apparent predisposing risk factors. The likelihood of epilepsy varies with the type of cerebral palsy, occurring in about 50–80% of children with hemiplegic or quadriplegic cerebral palsy, and in 20% of those with dystonic or diplegic cerebral palsy. For each type of cerebral palsy, the incidence of epilepsy is highest in those with the most severe learning difficulties.

Learning difficulties[80,81]

The risk of epilepsy increases with increasing severity of learning disability, being found in around 10% of children with mild learning difficulties, in about 40% of those with severe learning difficulties, and in up to 50% of children with autism when associated with significant learning difficulties.

There is a complex relationship between epilepsy and learning difficulties. Sometimes both have a common cause (e.g. genetic) but in other cases the epilepsy itself or very frequent and apparently subclinical epileptiform activity (spike and slow-wave activity) may be responsible for either temporary or permanent learning problems. The treatment of epilepsy may, in some cases, also contribute towards an impairment of a child's learning ability, and although it is important to try and control the epilepsy, multiple drug prescribing – and particularly using high doses – should be avoided. It is extremely unlikely that any child will gain additional seizure control, and without cognitive or behavioural side-effects, on three rather than two drugs; there is therefore little, if any, indication for using more than two drugs simultaneously. When epilepsy surgery is considered appropriate, the earlier it is undertaken, the greater will be the

opportunity for a child to benefit from any educational and general developmental support being offered, particularly for patients with mesial temporal lobe epilepsy (MTLE).

The genetics of epilepsy[82–85]

In 70–75% of children with epilepsy no cause will be found; a large proportion of these cases may have, or will subsequently be found to have, a genetic cause. Gene analysis is revealing that most of these epilepsies are due to mutations either in neurotransmitter receptors or in neuronal ion channels (channelopathies).[85] This is discussed in more detail in the following chapter.

Figures 10–20 *illustrate some of the more common abnormalities which are readily demonstrated by computed tomography, magnetic resonance or SPECT imaging.*

Figure 10
MRI scan (T2-weighted, axial image) of a 9-year-old girl with a grade 3 parieto-thalamic astrocytoma who presented with a 3-week history of frequent daily simple and complex partial seizures affecting only her right arm and face. Between seizures she had no neurological deficit.

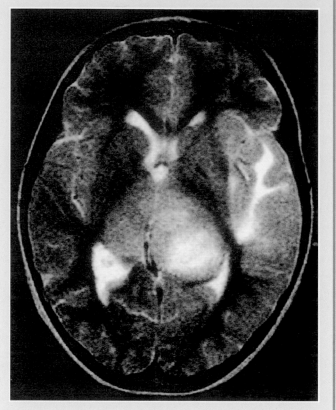

Figure 11
MRI scan (T2-weighted, axial image) of an 8-month-old boy with tuberous sclerosis who presented with a 4-week history of infantile spasms and irritability (scan shows subependymal nodules [protruding into the lateral ventricles] and multiple areas of high signal within the cerebral white matter – cortical tubers).

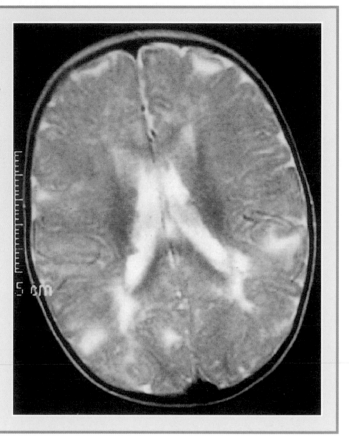

Figure 12
MRI scan (T2-weighted, axial image) of a 12-month-old boy with lissencephaly who presented with seizures from 7 weeks of age and subsequently demonstrated spastic quadriplegia, cortical visual impairment and almost no developmental progress (scan shows a smooth cerebral surface with minimal gyral formation and a thick cortical mantle).

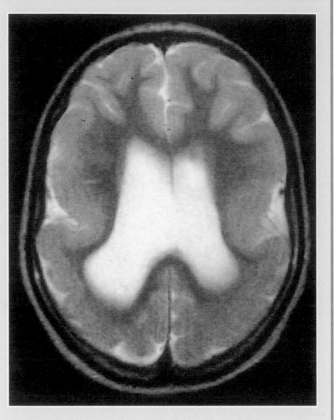

Figure 13
MRI scan (T2-weighted, magnified coronal image) of a 12-year-old girl showing a small and dysplastic left hippocampus who presented with drug-resistant complex partial and secondarily generalized seizures from 3 years of age.

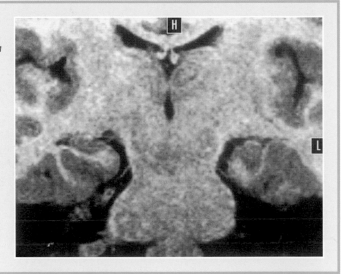

Figure 14
MRI scan (T1-weighted, coronal image) of a 15-year-old girl showing left-sided hippocampal atrophy without any mesial temporal sclerosis who presented with partial seizures from 10 years of age; she had experienced two prolonged 'febrile' seizure at 8 months of age.

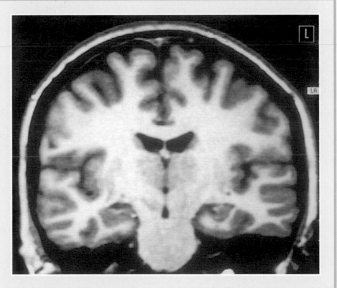

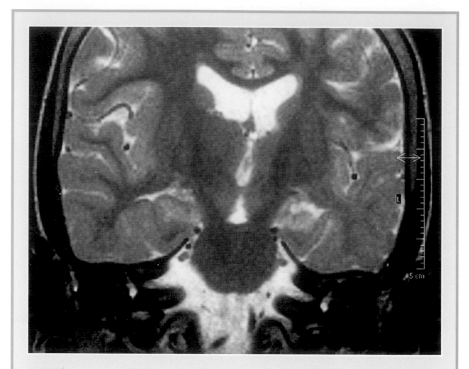

Figure 15
MRI scan (T2-weighted, coronal image) of a 13-year-old boy showing left mesial temporal sclerosis who presented with simple and complex partial seizures from 9 years of age; he had experienced a single prolonged tonic–clonic convulsion without fever at 5 months of age.

Figure 16
MRI scan (T2-weighted, axial image) of a 5-year-old girl showing a focal area of gliosis affecting the left frontal lobe which complicated a surgical procedure. She experienced frequent right-sided 'Jacksonian' motor and complex partial seizures (manifest as atypical absences).

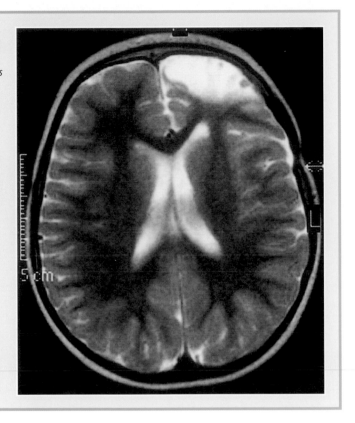

Figure 17
CT scan (axial image) of a 4-year-old boy showing a small and dysplastic left hemisphere, schizencephaly and an absent corpus callosum; he had a right hemiplegia, cortical visual impairment and frequent partial and generalized (tonic, atonic and tonic–clonic) seizures.

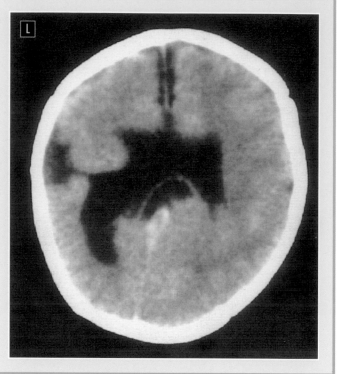

Figure 18
MRI scan (T2-weighted, axial image) showing extensive areas of high signal in the right parietal and posterior temporal cortex in a 9-year-old boy, consistent with herpes simplex encephalitis, who presented with a 3-day history of headache, pyrexia and brief seizures affecting his left arm and the left side of his face. CSF analysis showed a lymphocytosis. (NB: herpes simplex encephalitis more commonly affects the anterior temporal lobes.)

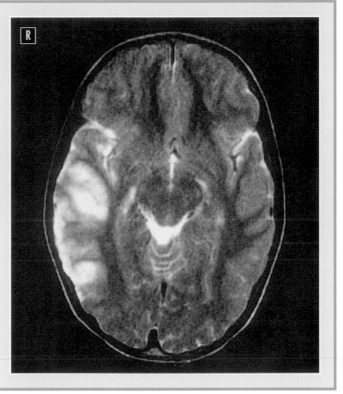

Figure 19
Interictal and ictal HMPAO-SPECT scans of an 8-year-old child with daily complex partial seizures with left mesial temporal sclerosis and left occipital lobe atrophy on MRI. The arrows show hypo-perfusion in the left temporal and left occipital regions on the interictal scan (a) and subtle hyper-perfusion in the left temporal lobe with no evidence of hyper-perfusion in the left occipital lobe on the ictal scan (b).

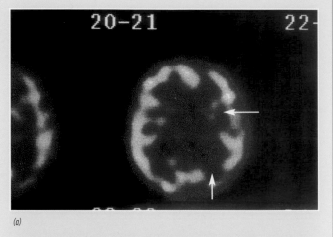

(a)

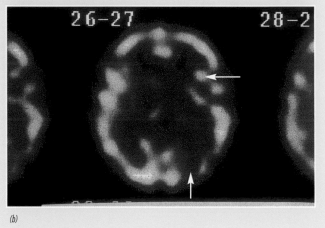

(b)

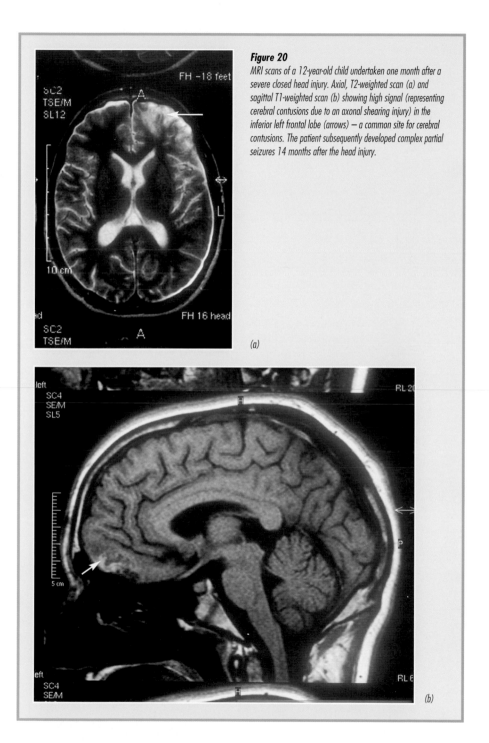

Figure 20
MRI scans of a 12-year-old child undertaken one month after a severe closed head injury. Axial, T2-weighted scan (a) and sagittal T1-weighted scan (b) showing high signal (representing cerebral contusions due to an axonal shearing injury) in the inferior left frontal lobe (arrows) – a common site for cerebral contusions. The patient subsequently developed complex partial seizures 14 months after the head injury.

(a)

(b)

Genetics of epilepsy

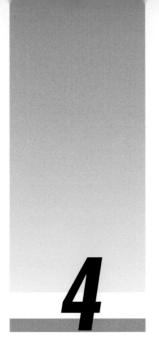

4

In 70–75% of children, no cause for the epilepsy will be found. Between 30% and 50% of these cases (i.e. ≥33% of all children with epilepsy) may have a genetic basis, particularly in those children who have primary generalized seizures. It is possible that benign familial neonatal convulsions may represent the youngest manifestation of a primary or idiopathic generalized epilepsy syndrome. Primary or idiopathic generalized epilepsies are usually inherited as an autosomal dominant trait.

Chromosomal localizations have been discovered for a large number of epilepsies or epilepsy syndromes and other disorders which include epilepsy as a common or prominent feature:[58]

Genetics of epilepsy – chromosomal localization

Epilepsy/epilepsy syndrome/disease	Chromosomal location
Benign familial neonatal convulsions	8q and 20q
Hyperekplexia	5q
Tuberous sclerosis complex 1	9q3.4
Tuberous sclerosis complex 2	16p13.3
Early infantile neuronal ceroid lipofuscinosis	1q
Late infantile neuronal ceroid lipofuscinosis ('Batten's disease')	11p15
Neurofibromatosis type 1	17q11.2
Miller–Dieker syndrome (characterized by lissencephaly)	17p
Wolf–Hirschhorn syndrome	4p16.3 deletion
Autosomal dominant nocturnal frontal lobe epilepsy	20q
Huntington's disease	4p
Partial epilepsies (including partial epilepsy with rolandic spikes)	10q2.3
Juvenile myoclonic epilepsy	6p and 15q
Progressive myoclonic epilepsy (Mediterranean and Baltic myoclonus and Unverricht–Lundborg disease)	21q
Generalized epilepsy and febrile seizures plus	9

Autosomal dominant nocturnal frontal lobe epilepsy (ADNFLE) is a relatively recently described epilepsy characterized by clusters of brief nocturnal motor seizures with hyperkinetic, tonic or dystonic movements.[44,45,88] Patients may often experience a brief aura and may remain aware and conscious throughout the attacks. Seizures tend to cluster with 4–12/night, and may be misdiagnosed as a benign sleep phenomenon (including night terrors or other parasomnia) or a psychiatric (i.e. pseudo- or non-epileptic attacks) or medical (e.g. obstructive sleep apnoea) disorder. The epilepsy usually begins in mid–late childhood and may persist throughout adult life. The interictal EEG is frequently normal and unhelpful, neuro-imaging is usually normal and carbamazepine or oxcarbazepine are generally effective in controlling the seizures. Other drugs effective against partial seizures may also be used (e.g. lamotrigine or topiramate).

There are numerous other disorders of which epilepsy is often a prominent feature, including:

- MERRF (**m**yoclonic **e**pilepsy and **r**agged **r**ed **f**ibres seen on muscle biopsy), caused by a maternally derived DNA point mutation (commonly 8344)

- MELAS (**m**itochondrial **e**ncephalopathy, **l**actic **a**cidosis and **s**troke-like episodes) in which children may present with or develop focal seizures and epilepsia partialis continua, caused by a maternally derived DNA point mutation (commonly 3234)

- Fragile X syndrome – nuclear-derived DNA mutation

- Down's syndrome – trisomy 21

- Other chromosomal disorders – trisomy 12 and ring chromosomes 14 and 20

Epilepsy is common in children with Fragile X syndrome, occurring in between

20% and 40%, and may include partial and generalized (all types) seizures. Seizures occur far less commonly in Down's syndrome (<10%) but almost half of these children will develop seizures in the first year of life, particularly infantile spasms, myoclonic and tonic–clonic seizures.

Progressive neuronal degeneration of childhood (PNDC), with or without liver disease (often called Alper's disease when the liver is involved), is a rare disorder, usually presenting in the first two or three years of life (but occasionally much later) with severe myoclonic seizures or epilepsia partialis continua, which may also be due to an inherited metabolic disorder, involving fatty acid oxidation and possibly mitochondrial in origin. In the past some children with this condition may have been falsely diagnosed as suffering and dying from sodium valproate-induced hepatoxicity.[89] Brain imaging with CT or MRI usually shows progressive and marked cerebral atrophy. Children usually die within 1–3 years of presentation.

Photosensitivity may also be genetically determined. It is a commonly occurring phenomenon, in association with the idiopathic generalized epilepsies, particularly in juvenile myoclonic epilepsy, and is twice as common in girls. The phenomenon is far less frequently seen in some partial (focal) epilepsies. Photosensitivity tends to develop between 10 and 16 years of age and usually resolves by the end of the second decade, although it may persist into middle age.

It is unlikely that the idiopathic generalized epilepsies are caused by single genes. Inheritance is more likely to be polygenic with the probability of additional seizure-modifying (facilitatory or inhibitory) genes or other 'influences' resulting from exogenous or environmental factors. Inheritance in this situation is said to be non-Mendelian or complex/multifactorial. 'Typical' examples of this type of inheritance are illustrated by the idiopathic generalized epilepsy syndromes of juvenile myoclonic epilepsy (JME) and childhood-onset absence epilepsy (CAE). It could reasonably have been expected that both may have the same genetic basis as both share a number of similar clinical features. However, this does not appear to be the case. Some (but importantly not all) families with JME have been linked to chromosome 6p, in contrast to, as yet, no families with CAE. More recently, the α-7 sub-unit of the neuronal nicotinic acetylcholine receptor gene, which lies on chromosome 15, has been implicated in other families with JME. Importantly, within an individual family, affected family members may have different types of epilepsy or epilepsy syndromes, including CAE or JME or epilepsy with grand mal on awakening – or even mesial temporal lobe epilepsy (a 'partial' epilepsy).

The occurrence of both generalized and partial epilepsies within a family could theoretically be explained by chance; however, if in the future it is shown that there is a clear genetic basis for generalized *and* partial epilepsies within the same individual family, this will clearly challenge the current dichotomy between the 'partial' and 'generalized' epilepsies.

Further evaluation and classification of the inheritance of the epilepsies is clearly important and is dependent on identifying 'pure' populations with specific syndromes, as well as developing further advances in molecular genetics. The resulting information should increase the understanding of the pathogenesis of the epilepsies, including the influence of environmental factors, its management (accurate genetic counselling and, possibly, the development of rational treatments, although this is currently somewhat speculative and has been discussed for the past decade) and even the prevention of specific disorders featuring difficult epilepsies (e.g. the neuronal ceroid lipofuscinoses and tuberous sclerosis).

Counselling in the more common epilepsies – particularly the idiopathic generalized epilepsies – is frequently requested by families. An empiric risk of epilepsy developing is 5–10% for children whose siblings or parents have one of these epilepsies (e.g. CAE, JME or epilepsy with grand mal on awakening); the risk is increased to at least 15–25% (if not greater) if both a parent and a sibling have one of these epilepsies. However, it is not possible to predict precisely what type of generalized epilepsy the child may develop, for reasons described above.

In benign partial epilepsy with centro-temporal (rolandic) spikes, the sibling of an affected child has a 10–15% risk of inheriting this epilepsy syndrome.

71

Neonatal seizures

5

The newborn period is the time of life with the highest
risk of seizures and epilepsy (*Figure 1*, page 4). This is
because of the relative lack of, and immature
development of, inhibitory neurotransmitters and their
pathways. This renders the immature brain relatively
'excitable' and more likely to seize. The newborn brain
is therefore more susceptible to a large number of
cerebral and systemic insults (which may be transient
or permanent). The precise incidence of neonatal
seizures is unclear, but is probably 1–3%; it is far greater
in those infants who have a high risk of developing
seizures, including those who have suffered an hypoxic–
ischaemic insult and those with a cerebral
malformation.

Diagnosis

The recognition of neonatal seizures may be difficult
and, as a consequence, they are both over- and under-
diagnosed. Neonates frequently demonstrate abnormal,
involuntary movements that are not epileptic. Normal
movements may also be mistaken for seizures.
Jitteriness and spontaneous clonus are the most
commonly misdiagnosed movements for epileptic
seizures.

Seizure types in the newborn infant are different from
those in older children.[90–93] Generalized tonic–clonic

seizures are rare (particularly in premature infants). Most seizures are subtle, myoclonic or clonic (predominantly partial or focal, including Jacksonian, but also generalized). The current classification, and relative frequency of neonatal seizures is shown in the box below.[90]

- Clonic
- Tonic
- Myoclonic
- Spasms
- Motor automatisms
- Autonomic events
- EEG seizures only
- Unclassified

1.	Subtle (30%)	— Bicycling (pedalling) or boxing movements Oral–buccal–lingual (chewing, swallowing or tongue-thrusting) Eye deviation (downwards or upwards) Apnoea
2.	Clonic (25%)	— Focal (one arm or leg) Multifocal (e.g. ipsilateral arm; contralateral leg) Jacksonian ('marching' or migrating distally → proximally)
3.	Myoclonic (20%)	— Focal Multifocal Generalized
4.	Tonic (20%)	— Generalized Focal

Subtle seizures are more common in premature infants. Subtle refers to their motor manifestation, and not to their underlying cause, which may be due to a severe cerebral insult, including hypoxia, meningo-encephalitis or cerebral dysgenesis. Although apnoea may represent a subtle seizure, it is rarely the only seizure type seen, and is more commonly due to some other cause (e.g. sepsis or 'apnoea of prematurity').

Tonic seizures are usually generalized (rather than focal), and may be the presenting sign of a periventricular haemorrhage (particularly in a pre-term infant).

This classification is not universally accepted, is being revised and is likely to be replaced with a new classification in the near future; the ILAE task force has not apparently considered neonatal seizures in its proposed new classification.[29] An abridged form of this classification is likely to be the following:

It cannot be over-emphasized that not all abnormal movements (particularly in pre-term infants) are seizures; clinical differentiation of seizure from non-seizure activity may be very difficult, and the following must be considered:

- Jitteriness (see below)

- Clonus (spontaneous or stimulus-sensitive)

- Fragmentary myoclonic jerks – multiple or single (may occur when awake, asleep or wakening from sleep)

- Roving, dysconjugate eye movements

- Oral (sucking, lip-puckering) movements

- 'Stretching'

- Benign neonatal sleep myoclonus

- Tonic reflex activity (manifestation of severe neurological damage)

- Hyperekplexia (see below)

Jitteriness: characteristically a movement phenomenon of the newborn (from a few hours to 1–2 weeks of age), is frequently confused with a seizure. Tremulousness is the predominant feature, although clonus may also occur. It differs from seizure activity in five ways:

1. It is unaccompanied by ocular phenomenon (eye fixation or deviation)

2. It is extremely sensitive to external stimuli

3. The dominant movement is tremor (the alternating movements are rhythmic, of equal rate and amplitude; in seizures the movements are clonic with a fast and slow component)

4. The fast, rhythmic movements of the limbs in jitteriness are usually stopped either by holding or by passively flexing the limb(s)

5. Autonomic changes are common in seizures, but not in jitteriness

Hyperekplexia:[94–98] (also known as 'startle disease' or 'congenital stiff-man syndrome') may present in the first few days or weeks of life with prolonged tonic spasms or an exaggerated startle response, often in response to unexpected auditory or tactile stimuli. Tapping the nose gently readily induces a 'startle', which does not 'habituate' or diminish/disappear with repeated taps. At rest the infants are hypertonic and may lie in the fetal position. Spontaneous nocturnal myoclonus and, later in infancy, epileptic seizures may occur. The tonic spasms are sudden, and may lead to apnoea and death. These spasms may be terminated by passively flexing the infant, particularly their neck or body. The pathogenesis is probably due to a channelopathy, inherited in an autosomal dominant pattern. Different mutations in the alpha 1 subunit of the inhibitory glycine receptor (*GLRA1*) gene have been identified in many affected families. These mutations result in a channelopathy that impairs the chloride channel function of inhibitory glycine receptors. This leads to an increased excitability in ponto-medullary neurons within the brainstem and abnormal spinal reciprocal inhibition. The gene has been mapped to chromosome 5q. There are almost certainly additional mutations in the inhibitory receptor genes mapping to different chromosomes and with different patterns of inheritance. The phenomenon may diminish or disappear by 2–3 years of age, although the epileptic seizures (if present) may persist. Clonazepam or clobazam are of benefit for the tonic spasms and exaggerated startle responses.

EEG (particularly prolonged with simultaneous video-recording of the clinical episodes and abnormal movements) may resolve some of the difficulty or uncertainty and 'confirm' (or refute) whether the infant is having seizures. However, there is frequently an element of 'electroclinical dissociation' in which the electroencephalographic seizures have an inconstant relationship with clinical seizures.

Seizure type		EEG correlation	
		common	*uncommon*
Subtle		+/−	+/−
Myoclonic:	generalized	+	
	focal		+
Clonic:	multifocal	+	
	focal	+	
Tonic	generalized		+

The absence of epileptic discharges on a scalp EEG does not necessarily exclude a clinical epileptic seizure; the seizure may be arising from subcortical (limbic,

diencephalic, brainstem) structures. Clearly it may be difficult to differentiate 'normal' and common brainstem release phenomena (e.g. benign neonatal sleep myoclonus) from a seizure originating from within the brainstem – however, brainstem seizures are very uncommon.

Once the diagnosis of epileptic seizures has been established, the next step is to identify the cause. In contrast to the case with older children, but similar to that with adults, an underlying cause is often discovered.

Aetiology and investigation

It is important to realize that the majority of seizures occurring in the newborn period are symptomatic or cryptogenic; very few (approximately 5%) are idiopathic. The timing of onset of seizures is closely related to their cause *(Figure 21 and Table 9)*.

Table 9
Aetiology and onset of neonatal seizures.

Within 24 hours of birth
Perinatal asphyxia (hypoxic–ischaemic encephalopathy)
Periventricular haemorrhage
Hypoglycaemia
Sepsis, including meningitis
Congenital infection (herpes simplex, rubella, cytomegalovirus, toxoplasmosis, HIV)
Laceration of tentorium of falx (perinatal trauma)
Cerebral malformation (dysgenesis)
Drug withdrawal (maternal use of alcohol, hypnotics, barbiturates)
Pyridoxine (vitamin B6) dependency
Maternal use of local anaesthetic agents (during labour and delivery)

Continued

Table 9 *Continued*

At 24–72 hours of age
As for within 24 hours, plus: Metabolic disorders (see below) Benign neonatal convulsions – familial (autosomal dominant) 　　　　　　　　　　　　　　　　　　　– sporadic Hypocalcaemia Cerebral contusion with subdural haemorrhage Kernicterus (hyperbilirubinaemia)
At 1 week
Cerebral malformation (dysgenesis) Herpes simplex (acquired) Sepsis Ketotic hyperglycinaemia; maple syrup urine disease Metabolic disorders (see later)

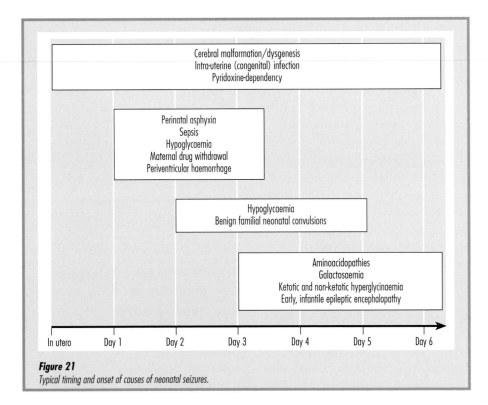

Figure 21
Typical timing and onset of causes of neonatal seizures.

Metabolic disorders causing neonatal seizures (excluding impairment of glucose, sodium, calcium and magnesium)[59,60]

Adrenoleucodystrophy (neonatal; usually x-linked)

Biotinidase deficiency

Folinic acid-responsive neonatal seizures

Galactosaemia

Gaucher's disease

Hyperammonaemia (often associated with aminoacidopathy)

Maple syrup urine disease

Mitochondrial cytopathy

Multiple carboxylase deficiency

Niemann–Pick disease

Non-ketotic and ketotic hyperglycinaemia

Organic acidaemias

Pyridoxine dependency

Pyruvate dehydrogenase complex deficiency

Sulphite oxidase and molybdenum co-factor deficiencies

Urea cycle disorders

Zellweger's syndrome (peroxisosomal disorder)

In the most common cause (hypoxic–ischaemic encephalopathy), seizures tend to develop in the first 6–24 hours of life, and are severe, frequent and even continuous; seizures may be tonic, clonic (usually multifocal) and subtle. This aetiology is responsible for approximately 40–50% of all neonatal seizures, particularly in term neonates. In neonates born prematurely, intraventricular/intraparenchymal haemorrhage is the most common cause of neonatal seizures.

In most cases the underlying cause can be determined from the perinatal (including pregnancy) and birth history, the family history, the early clinical course and the neurological/physical examination.

An initial 'screen' should include:

- *Blood glucose, calcium, magnesium, electrolytes and acid–base status*
- *Full blood count and blood film examination*
- *Cerebrospinal fluid analysis (glucose, protein, cell count)*
- *Cultures of blood, CSF, urine and faeces*
- *Cranial ultrasonography*

Further investigations should be performed depending upon the clinical situation:[59,60]

- *Blood ammonia, lactate, urate and liver enzymes*
- *Blood and urine amino acids; urinary organic acids*
- *Urine-reducing substances*
- *'TORCH' and other antibody studies (for congenital infections)*
- *Diagnostic use of pyridoxine (vitamin B6)*
- *CT of head (for cerebral malformations/dysgenesis)*

CT may not reveal subtle dysgenesis (such as heterotopic grey matter) or abnormal patterns of myelination until the infant is at least six months of age, if not older when myelination is complete (2–3 yrs); MRI may be more sensitive. However, early CT (within the first few weeks of life) should reveal major cerebral malformations (e.g. lissencephaly, schizencephaly and holoprosencephaly) and evidence of a moderate or severe hypoxic–ischaemic cerebral insult.

It is possible that viral infections, sustained at any time during fetal life and not confined to rubella, CMV or herpes simplex type 1, may represent a significant cause of neonatal seizures[64] This should justify a more detailed search for a viral aetiology, including CSF analysis (white cell count, viral-specific IgG antibody levels etc.) and polymerase chain reaction (PCR) studies, particularly in the absence of an obvious hypoxic, structural or biochemical cause for the seizures.

Treatment[99]

There are a number of issues to consider when treating neonatal seizures:

- *The most important is to identify and where possible correct any underlying metabolic/biochemical disorder (e.g. hypocalcaemia, hypoglycaemia, etc.)*
- *Other obvious causes should be excluded (e.g. maternal drug withdrawal, intracerebral/periventricular haemorrhage, cerebral dysgenesis)*
- *Pyridoxine (vitamin B6) should be given if early seizures are resistant to 'conventional' anticonvulsant therapy and if there is no obvious cause for the seizures[100]*
- *Not every infant will necessarily need to be treated with an anticonvulsant*
- *It is important to maintain homeostasis (particularly blood pressure and oxygen and glucose supplies) during repeated or prolonged convulsions*
- *Hypoxia, hypoglycaemia and hypotension/hypertension may contribute significantly in causing additional secondary neuronal damage, which may further increase the risk of developing 'late' epilepsy*

Although there may be some agreement in treating repeated seizures (occurring more than two or three times an hour) or prolonged seizures (lasting more than 3–5 minutes), with an anticonvulsant, there is less agreement in using one of these drugs in treating far less frequent or far briefer seizures.[99]

A similar dilemma exists when deciding what seizure types should be treated; tonic, clonic and 'subtle' seizures should demand more 'aggressive' anticonvulsant treatment than isolated myoclonic seizures, but this must also be correlated with the frequency and duration of the seizures.

Debate also exists over the EEG findings, particularly in view of the electroclinical dissociation between the clinical seizures and EEG appearances. There is no rational argument for aiming to suppress all abnormal paroxysmal activity on the EEG, firstly as this is unlikely to be successful and secondly as in doing so the infant may be over-sedated and exposed to the greater risk of drug toxicity. Finally, there is as yet no convincing evidence that treating purely electrical seizures on the EEG either significantly influences or improves the long-term neurodevelopmental outcome of these infants. Further information is clearly needed to try and clarify this important issue.

The 'optimal' duration of treatment with an anticonvulsant after neonatal seizures is also unclear. The risk of recurrent seizures outside the neonatal period and during the first year of life following a week of anticonvulsant treatment is generally low (<10%) but will depend on the cause.

In view of this it would seem reasonable to continue an antiepileptic drug for only one or two weeks after the apparent cessation of any neonatal seizures – and this is the authors' usual practice. Some clinicians recommend withdrawing the anticonvulsant when the infant is neurologically 'normal'; this is not entirely logical or necessarily appropriate as a significant number of infants will remain neurologically and developmentally abnormal outside the neonatal period but not develop further seizures. It would

seem more appropriate to re-start antiepileptic medication only if an infant developed later epilepsy.

The antiepileptic drugs most frequently used in the treatment of neonatal seizures include:

Lorazepam; clonazepam (the latter with a loading dose of 100–300 μg/kg ± infusion at 10–30 μg/kg/h);

Diazepam (intravenous; rarely rectal)

Phenobarbitone (intravenous; oral)

Phenytoin (intravenous; oral)

Paraldehyde (rectal or intravenous infusion of a 5% solution at 0.5–3 ml/kg/h)

Lignocaine

Carbamazepine; vigabatrin (oral)

The benzodiazepines (preferably lorazepam (0.05–0.1 mg/kg) or clonazepam) are useful for repeated or prolonged seizures and are probably the drugs of choice for treating seizures that are likely to be a transient phenomenon.

Phenobarbitone is the most commonly used antiepileptic drug for neonatal seizures and for short-term use is the preferred drug. There is also some evidence that using phenobarbitone *before* seizures develop may be 'neuro-protective' in reducing the incidence of seizures and even 'improving' the long-term prognosis in neonates who have experienced hypoxic–ischaemic encephalopathy.[101,102] The intravenous loading dose is usually 20 mg/kg although occasionally in refractory and prolonged seizures (including status epilepticus) higher doses of 30–50 mg/kg may be required. The usual maintenance dose is 3–8 mg/kg/day. However, there is evidence that phenobarbitone may not necessarily improve the abnormal EEGs in some neonates,[101] although whether this is clinically important is unclear for reasons already discussed.

Phenytoin is also effective;[103] its main advantage is its lack of respiratory depression, although it may cause a cardiac arrhythmia or hypotension (or both) if the loading dose is infused too rapidly. The 'usual' loading dose is 15–18 mg/kg, with a maintenance dose of 5–15 mg/kg/day (given either 8- or 12-hourly) but occasionally higher doses (20–30 mg/kg/day) may be required to maintain 'therapeutic' blood levels and improve seizure control. The metabolism of phenytoin in the neonate is very unpredictable, particularly if other drugs are being used (including antibiotics), and this makes the drug somewhat difficult to use and necessitates frequent serum monitoring to prevent toxicity. Ideally, phenytoin should not be used outside the neonatal period and infancy.

The combination of phenobarbitone and phenytoin may occasionally be more effective in controlling seizures than when either drug is used alone.

If it is felt necessary to continue using an antiepileptic drug beyond the neonatal period, drugs such as carbamazepine, vigabatrin or lamotrigine should be used as alternatives to phenobarbitone/phenytoin. Sodium valproate should either be avoided or used with caution at this age in view of any possible underlying metabolic/liver disorder that may be responsible for/contribute to the hepatotoxicity which has been reported with this drug. The children who appear to be most at risk of liver failure in association with the use of sodium valproate are those with the following features: less than 3 years of age with severe epilepsy (including myoclonic seizures), global and usually severe developmental delay for which no cause has been found and receiving at least two antiepileptic drugs.

Prognosis

A number of factors will influence and determine the outcome of neonates with seizures:

- Aetiology of seizures (probably the most important factor)
- Type or degree of associated brain injury
- Gestational (and therefore maturational) age of the infant
- Seizure type
- Seizure frequency (particularly if repeated and in clusters)
- Seizure duration

The prognosis for infants with seizures in the neonatal period has improved over the past 10–15 years, largely due to advances in neonatal intensive care and support. Outcome is poorest in:

- Very small infants (small for gestational age or premature or both – **Table 10**)

- Seizures occurring and frequent in the first 72 hours of life

- Seizures due to hypoxic–ischaemic encephalopathy

- Seizures due to periventricular haemorrhage

- Seizures due to hypoglycaemia

- Seizures due to cerebral dysgenesis

- Markedly abnormal background activity on interictal EEG

Structural and even functional imaging may also provide some predictive information: e.g. the 'acute reversal sign'

seen on CT is a characteristic feature of a severe hypoxic–ischaemic encephalopathy, and heralds a very poor outcome.

These infants frequently develop infantile spasms (West's syndrome), often from as young as 3 or 4 months of age, and the spasms are extremely resistant to all antiepileptic drugs including vigabatrin and steroids; in the authors' experience nitrazepam and topiramate seem to offer the most effective treatments in this specific group.

Table 10
Prognosis of neonatal seizures in relation to maturity. (From Volpe 1995.)[90]

Maturity	Outcome		
	Normal	**Dead**	**CNS sequelae**
Term (>2500 g)	60%	19%	21%
Pre-term (<2500 g)	35%	37%	28%
Pre-term (<1500 g)	19%	58%	23%

Outstanding issues

1. Inadequate data indicating whether neonatal seizures produce cerebral damage or are completely 'harmless'; although it is unlikely that repeated persistent seizures are entirely 'harmless', it is likely that the aetiology of the seizures is as or more important than the seizures themselves.

2. It is not always clear which infants require maintenance antiepileptic drug therapy

3. The duration of antiepileptic drug therapy is not known – particularly in infants who become seizure-free outside the newborn period

4. Does the early use of antiepileptic drug therapy influence the development of, and specifically prevent, later epilepsy?

5. There is almost no information on the effects of antiepileptic drugs on the developing brain, and particularly on the excitatory and inhibitory neurotransmitters and their relevant receptors. The reported association of phenytoin and irreversible cerebellar damage requires further evaluation

Febrile seizures

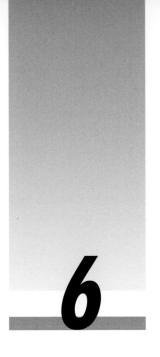

A febrile seizure is generally and practically defined as 'a convulsion (or seizure) with fever in children aged between 6 months and 5 years without evidence of meningitis or encephalitis'.

Some authors believe that children who are defined as having a febrile seizure must be normal neurologically and developmentally, while others consider that minor neurological dysfunction or 'mild' developmental delay is acceptable. Most would agree that a child with a chronic brain disorder (including established epilepsy) could not have a febrile convulsion.[104] Finally, some authors would not accept that febrile seizures are a distinct entity, but would consider them a form of epilepsy. These marked differences of opinion emphasize the difficulties in defining what precisely does, and does not, constitute a febrile seizure.

Febrile seizures are common, occurring in 2–4% of children between 6 months and 5 years, with a peak at 18 months to 3 years. They can be classified into:

Simple: which represent approximately 75% of all febrile seizures and are manifest by a generalized onset, tonic–clonic seizure lasting less than 15 minutes with no post-ictal neurological deficit or sequelae;

Complex (perhaps more appropriately described as 'complicated' to avoid confusion with 'complex' partial seizures): accounting for 25% and characterized by either a focal onset (or a persisting focal convulsion), repeated during the same febrile episode, prolonged (lasting over 15 minutes, including status epilepticus) or followed by a neurological deficit (including a Todd's paresis).

Generally, simple febrile convulsions tend to be associated with a better and complicated with a worse prognosis with regard to 'late epilepsy' and developmental status; however, this does not necessarily imply a causal relationship.

The risk of a child having a febrile seizure is:

> • *40–50% if a sibling and one parent had febrile seizures*
> • *10% if a sibling had febrile seizures*
> • *15% if a parent had febrile seizures*
> • *0–5% if a parent has/had afebrile seizures (epilepsy)*
> • *5–10% if a sibling has/had afebrile seizures (epilepsy)*

The precise mode of inheritance is unclear, but is generally believed to be either autosomal dominant with reduced penetrance and variable expression or, as is more likely, polygenic. Thirty per cent of children who have had one febrile convulsion will have a second, and 1 in 3 of these will have a third febrile seizure.

Most recurrences are complicated (complex) in type.

Recent advances in neuroradiology (high-resolution MRI) and molecular genetics have confirmed that the concept of what does and does not constitute a 'febrile seizure' needs revision – and there should be a re-evaluation of the controversial and at times uncomfortable relationship between 'febrile' seizures and later epilepsy:

• The demonstration of structural abnormalities, including cortical dysplasia, neuronal migration abnormalities (e.g. grey matter heterotopia) and sclerosis in the temporal, and to a lesser extent, the frontal lobes on MRI undertaken after only one or two 'febrile' seizures[105,106] – and before recurrent and prolonged febrile seizures can cause further hypothetical damage within the hippocampus of the temporal lobe.
• The identification of a new syndrome of generalized epilepsy and febrile seizures 'plus' (GEFS+).[41,107] This syndrome may initially present with febrile seizures in the first two years of life, before the development of generalized tonic–clonic seizures in later childhood or early adult life. Other family members with the same genetic syndrome can experience other seizure types, including myoclonic, atonic and partial seizures without a prior history of partial seizures as well as 'febrile' seizures in late childhood. The most common

pattern of inheritance is autosomal dominant with at least two abnormal genes on chromosomes 2 and 9.

The risk of a child with febrile seizures developing afebrile seizures (epilepsy) has received considerable attention but remains unclear. Most population- or community- (rather than hospital-) based studies suggest that this risk is between 2% and 5%. No definite factor or factors have been identified which will predict whether epilepsy will develop; complicated febrile seizures (even febrile status epilepticus) may be followed by epileptic seizures, but this is not invariable, and is not necessarily 'cause-and-effect'.[108–111] It is likely that in some children whose first complicated (complex) seizure with fever represents the earliest manifestation of their epilepsy, the co-occurrence of the fever and the seizure is entirely coincidental. The alleged damage caused by a complicated febrile seizure is mesial temporal (hippocampal) sclerosis (MTS).[75,76,109] Although there may be an apparent association, this again is not necessarily causative, and, importantly, MTS may be seen in children (and adults) who have never experienced a febrile seizure.[109,111] An alternative hypothesis is that there is an underlying developmental or acquired (in the neonatal/perinatal period) abnormality that may be responsible for a complicated seizure, which may have been simply triggered by a febrile illness.[75,76] It is possible that this complicated seizure may then produce further damage (possibly by focal hypoxic/ischaemic changes), but whether this actually occurs is unclear.[112] This hypothesis could be tested by early

(following a first complicated 'febrile' seizure), and long-term serial structural (MRI)[105] and functional (SPECT) imaging to document any early and evolving hippocampal atrophy. The role of other factors that may make children more susceptible to febrile seizures including interleukins and cytokines requires further evaluation.

Although *by definition* children as young as 6 months of age may have febrile seizures, the authors would not initially accept the diagnosis in infants less than 1 year of age, and would consider the following diagnoses first, and, where there is a high index of suspicion, undertake the appropriate investigations:

- *Meningitis/encephalitis*
- *Metabolic disorder*
- *Cerebral dysgenesis*

Clearly the number and type of investigations undertaken would depend upon the age of the infant and whether the 'febrile' seizure was 'simple' or 'complicated': e.g. one or more (recurrent) prolonged, predominantly focal, febrile seizure in a 6- or 8-month-old infant would justify at least the exclusion of meningitis by CSF analysis as well as urine culture and neuroimaging (preferably by MRI) to exclude (or demonstrate) a structural abnormality. In contrast, a simple febrile seizure in a 2- or 3-year-old child with an obvious ear infection probably needs no investigation. EEGs are rarely if ever of any use, even in complicated febrile seizures.

The acute management of children with febrile seizures includes ensuring that the airway is clear (and other first-aid measures). If prolonged, either intravenous (0.4–0.5 mg/kg) or rectal (0.4–0.5 mg/kg) diazepam is used to stop the convulsion. Lorazepam is an alternative (see Chapter 12 on Status epilepticus, page 137). Rectal diazepam administered at home may be used to both terminate seizures in infants and young children who have a low threshold of experiencing recurrent and prolonged seizures and also to prevent seizures from occurring (if given early enough) in any febrile illness – particularly in those children who have a low threshold for having complicated febrile seizures. Parents must receive appropriate counselling and advice about what febrile seizures are, and how to manage subsequent ones, including when and how to use rectal diazepam.

Importantly, prophylaxis with a maintenance oral antiepileptic drug (sodium valproate, carbamazepine or phenobarbitone) has not been shown to reduce significantly either the rate of recurrence of febrile seizures or, arguably more importantly, the development of subsequent epilepsy. Therefore, prophylactic long-term, oral use of an antiepileptic drug is not recommended.

Epilepsy in adolescence

Epilepsy is the most common neurological disorder of adolescence.[113] Epilepsy accounted for over 60% of all neurological problems in one American adolescent clinic,[114] and in another study of epilepsy in children the prevalence was found to be almost 9/1000 in children aged 15 years.[115]

For a teenager developing a first epileptic seizure, the incidence is approximately 75 per 100 000.

The prevalence of epilepsy in the teenage years is 6–7/1000.

Epilepsy starting in childhood frequently persists through adolescence and into adult life. Idiopathic generalized epilepsy (typically JME and epilepsy with grand mal on waking) and symptomatic partial epilepsy may begin at this age.[116] The range of epilepsies and epilepsy syndromes that may be encountered in adolescence include:

- *Idiopathic generalized*
  - *juvenile absence*
  - *juvenile myoclonic*
  - *epilepsy with grand mal on waking*
  - *reflex (including photosensitive, reading and eating) epilepsies*
- *Secondary (symptomatic) generalized*
- *Idiopathic partial (focal)*
  - *benign rolandic*
  - *benign occipital*
  - *primary reading epilepsy*
  - *benign focal epileptic seizures of teenagers/adolescence*
- *Secondary (symptomatic) partial*
- *Mesial temporal epilepsy*
- *Progressive myoclonic epilepsies*
- *Unclassified (partial or generalized)*

Causes of epilepsy in the adolescent include brain tumours (which, though rare, occur more commonly than in younger children, particularly supratentorially) and temporal lobe pathology, which is not necessarily preceded by earlier 'febrile seizures'. Other causes include substance abuse and as a sequel to head injuries.

Mesial temporal epilepsy (MTE) is a specific epilepsy that is frequently diagnosed in adolescence or early adult life, and, importantly, may well be progressive.[42,112] A characteristic history is of prolonged febrile or afebrile seizures occurring between 6 and 18 months of age, followed by simple partial sensory seizures from 5 to 9 years of age ('auras') that may or may not be recognized as seizures (because the children may not be able to accurately describe what they are feeling or what is happening to them). Between 10 and 16 years of age complex partial seizures with or without secondary generalized tonic–clonic seizures develop – and it may only be at this age that epilepsy is diagnosed. Patients also start to experience memory difficulties that may be progressive, and behavioural changes may occur. From 20 years of age seizures are usually refractory and patients may develop more overt psychopathology, including psychosis and social withdrawal. High-resolution MRI will usually demonstrate hippocampal atrophy and mesial temporal sclerosis as early as 8 or 9 years of age – although sometimes only later. Temporal lobe surgery has potentially a 75–80% chance of cure, providing all investigations are concordant for a single epileptogenic focus. In view of the progressive nature of MTE and the potential impressive cure rate, resective surgery must be considered sooner rather than later.

It is also important to realize that seizure type or frequency (or both) may change in adolescence as a result of many factors, including:

- *The natural history of the specific epilepsy/epilepsy syndrome*
- *The influence of age, including puberty and menarche (catamenial seizures), may also develop at this age*

- The effects of an erratic life-style (particularly sleep-deprivation and the use/abuse of alcohol or recreational drugs)
- Poor compliance with antiepileptic medication
- The development of photosensitivity as an age-dependent phenomenon (which may 'present' as the first epileptic seizure)

The differential diagnosis of seizures at this age is rather different than in earlier childhood, and includes the following:

- Syncope (vasovagal) attacks
- Migraine
- Non-epileptic attack disorder ('pseudo-epileptic seizures') – these are more likely to develop in a teenager who has had/is having genuine epileptic seizures, rather than in isolation)
- 'Group hysteria'; panic attacks and hyperventilation
- Substance abuse, particularly with cocaine, heroin or ecstasy (i.e. provoked epileptic seizure)
- Cardiac arrhythmia (specifically the prolonged QT interval syndrome and Wolff–Parkinson–White syndrome)
- An evolving neurodegenerative disorder (e.g. sub-acute sclerosing panencephalitis [SSPE], Lafora body disease, juvenile Huntington's disease, etc.)

The investigation of epilepsy in the teenager will depend upon the considered differential diagnosis, seizure type, neurological findings, epilepsy syndrome and likely cause.

The management of the teenager who has epilepsy is important, but is frequently inadequate. There are numerous specific issues and concerns unique to this age group, particularly regarding independence, which must be addressed to allow the teenager to pass successfully from childhood to maturity:[117–119]

- The prognosis of the epilepsy and which drug to use
- Whether to continue/discontinue treatment
- Whether to continue in further education
- Whether and how to apply for a job, and which job/career
- Relationships with family and friends
- Choices over leisure activities and driving
- Concern over alcohol, recreational drugs and sexual intercourse and how these might affect their epilepsy – and interact with their antiepileptic medication
- Decisions regarding pregnancy (including the effects of drugs on the fetus), contraception and the risks of passing epilepsy on to their children

Which drug to use: this largely depends on the seizure-type, the specific epilepsy syndrome and the side-effect profile of the drug. Teenage girls frequently stop taking sodium valproate because of weight gain (due to an increased appetite), hair loss and menstrual irregularities (including amenorrhoea and polycystic ovaries); lamotrigine may be preferable in this situation, particularly in the idiopathic generalized epilepsy syndromes, including epilepsy with 'grand mal' on waking and JME (*however, it is the authors' experience that lamotrigine may not be as effective as sodium valproate in controlling all the seizure types in JME*). Phenytoin and phenobarbitone should be avoided for obvious reasons (cosmetic and cognitive side-effects), but also as barbiturates (with or without alcohol) are one of the most frequently taken 'overdoses' in suicide and parasuicide, which are not rare events at this age.

All teenagers who present with a first or second tonic–clonic seizure **must** be specifically asked whether they also have jerks (myoclonic seizures), particularly in the first few hours after waking or episodes of 'blanking-out' or 'trances' (absence seizures). If the teenager does have myoclonic or absence seizures (or both) then sodium valproate or possibly lamotrigine should be used and carbamazepine must be avoided. Carbamazepine will typically exacerbate myoclonic and absence seizures and may even induce myoclonic or absence status in these teenagers. Phenytoin has a similar effect to carbamazepine and – because of its cosmetic side-effects and difficult metabolism – should also be avoided.

Discontinuing medication: this depends on the epilepsy syndrome, seizure control and the individual. It is important to give accurate advice on the risk of relapse if drugs are withdrawn, so that the teenager/family can make an informed decision.

Some generalized epilepsy syndromes, particularly JME, are associated with a high rate of relapse (at least 60%) if medication is withdrawn. The decision to withdraw must also consider other factors:

- *Whether the teenager is about to take an important examination, start a job or go abroad*

- *That a single seizure **of any type** (during or after drug withdrawal) may prevent the application for, or cause the loss of, a driving licence, and subsequently the loss of a job if the job is dependent on driving*

- *That there is no guarantee that seizures will or will not relapse*

- *That seizure control may, rarely, be more difficult to regain when the antiepileptic drug is reintroduced following a relapse*

- *That the antiepileptic drug must not be stopped suddenly, but gradually over a minimum of 6 or 8 weeks*

Non-compliance with antiepileptic medication is the most common cause of loss of, or poor, seizure control, including status epilepticus, in the teenager with epilepsy.

Specific issues: for teenage girls contraception and pregnancy are clearly very important issues. In pregnancy one third of women will experience a deterioration in seizure control, a third will experience an improvement and the remaining third no significant change. In certain situations (particularly if the teenager is accompanied by her boyfriend rather than by her parents), it is often prudent to raise the issue of pregnancy and contraception, as the teenage girl may be unaware of this as a potential problem or may be reluctant to initiate the discussion herself. The importance of pre-conception discussion and planning with medical staff should be emphasized, particularly in specific areas:

- *Optimize seizure control*
- *Use a single antiepileptic drug in the lowest effective dose wherever possible*
- *Avoid high peak blood levels of antiepileptic drugs; it would be wise to avoid slow or sustained-release preparations of drugs (which may be given once a day) and give the standard preparation twice or even three times a day)*
- *Folate supplements (a minimum of 0.4, and a maximum of 4–5 mg/day) should be given before and during pregnancy (ideally, folate supplements should be taken in any young woman with epilepsy who is sexually active)*
- *Early antenatal 'booking' and regular monitoring throughout pregnancy, preferably with access to a specialist fetal centre and 'state-of-the-art' fetal ultrasonography*

The choice of antiepileptic drug in the teenage girl is clearly important. Sodium valproate is known to increase the risk of neural tube defects (usually thoracic) at least tenfold up to 2% as well as being associated with the 'fetal valproate syndrome', which may occur in at least 5–10% of infants born to women taking sodium valproate during the first half of pregnancy. The 'syndrome' is characterized by certain facial features (including hypoplasia of the medial part of the eyebrows, a thin upper lip, absent/shallow philtrum and anteverted nostrils), other but less frequent anomalies (e.g. hypospadias and radial aplasia) and neurodevelopmental difficulties. Recent evidence has suggested that some antiepileptic drugs (particularly sodium valproate) may have an additional adverse effect on the child's development and specifically speech and language development and later cognitive functioning.[120] These are said to occur in the absence of any major congenital malformation or even minor, dysmorphic features. However, it is possible that these specific neurodevelopmental effects may reflect a cumulative or additive effect of not just the antiepileptic medication, but also risks from epilepsy, a genetic susceptibility and a familial history of learning difficulties. The results of collaborative national and international prospective research, with follow-up from birth into primary and secondary school (and beyond), should hopefully clarify this important issue. Carbamazepine also carries an increased risk of both neural tube defects (1% risk) and microcephaly. In view of these known teratogenic effects many clinicians are advocating that in teenage girls or young women of child-bearing potential who present with epilepsy, drugs such as gabapentin or lamotrigine should be the antiepileptic drugs of choice. However, this is based on relatively limited pregnancy data with these drugs and it must be realized that these 'newer' and apparently safer drugs do not yet have a licence for use in pregnancy.

Contraception is also an important issue – both the choice of contraception and, more specifically, the oral contraceptive, the most commonly used method. Certain antiepileptic drugs (e.g. carbamazepine, phenytoin, phenobarbitone and topiramate) may reduce the effectiveness of the oral contraceptive, thereby necessitating a higher strength (of the oestrogen content) of pill to ensure safe contraception. This effect is not seen or recognized with sodium valproate, gabapentin, lamotrigine, levetiracetam or vigabatrin.

Pregnancy is clearly an important issue – including for teenagers – particularly as up to 40% or 50% of pregnancies are unplanned and an increasing number of these unplanned pregnancies are in teenagers. The UK currently has the highest teenage pregnancy rate in Europe. Ideally, all women of childbearing age should be offered early pre-conception counselling so that the pregnancy can be planned with optimal management of the epilepsy. These women should receive folate supplementation as soon as they become sexually active, irrespective of whether a family is planned. This is because a missed menstrual cycle is usually not noticed until at least the 15th day post-conception and the risk of teratogenicity is greatest in the first trimester of pregnancy. Teratogenic sensitivity is greatest at 3–4 weeks for neural tube defects, 4–8 weeks for heart defects and 6–10 weeks for oro-facial cleft defects.[121,122]

There are also significant risks to the fetus if the woman has tonic–clonic seizures, including from the physical effects of falling (in a tonic–clonic or myoclonic seizure), as a consequence of hypoxic–ischaemic damage during a prolonged tonic–clonic seizure (i.e. status epilepticus) and also during delivery.

- During pregnancy, seizure control is generally unchanged in 1/3, improves in 1/3 and deteriorates in 1/3

- At constant drug dosage, the plasma levels of most antiepileptic drugs tend to fall during pregnancy (usually by week 10–12) and return to previous levels after pregnancy (usually by week 4–6). Decreased plasma levels may not necessarily be of any clinical significance. 'Routine' blood level monitoring is therefore not necessary

- Changes to antiepileptic medication should be made either **before** any pregnancy is planned or **after** the pregnancy

- A tonic–clonic seizure occurs during labour in 1–2% of women with epilepsy

- A tonic–clonic seizure occurs within the first 24 hours after delivery in 1–2%

Catamenial epilepsy is the exacerbation or restricted occurrence of seizures (usually generalized tonic–clonic or myoclonic seizures) just before or during menstruation. This may reflect hormonal changes, fluid retention and (in those already taking an antiepileptic drug), altered pharmacokinetics. Treatment may include the following:

- Temporarily increasing the dose of any maintenance antiepileptic drug 5–7 days before menses are due, and continuing for the duration of menstruation

- Using acetazolamide 250 mg or 500 mg daily beginning 5–7 days prior to the expected onset of menses, and continuing throughout menstruation

- Using clobazam, 10–20 mg daily beginning 2–4 days prior to the expected onset of menses, and continuing for the next 4–5 days

Career opportunities: this is frequently a very difficult but clearly important area and one that causes teenagers and young adults some confusion and considerable anxiety; not infrequently this is because their doctor (general practitioner [GP] or hospital consultant) gives inaccurate advice. Although there are clear limitations in employment opportunities for people with epilepsy, these are few and legislation does exist for providing special employment services – as in the 1995 Disabilities Discrimination Act. Teenagers can find further information from their local Disability Resettlement Officer (see Chapter 13 on the Impact of epilepsy for further details).

When completing a job application form it is the authors' usual practice to advise young people that the medical section of the first application form be left blank. The disclosure of epilepsy on the initial application form may serve to eliminate teenagers from any consideration of the job, irrespective of their qualifications or previous experience. However, if a firm offer of a job is made (either at interview or by letter), then epilepsy must then be disclosed and potential employers should also be given the name and address of the relevant hospital consultant.

Independence: The adolescent often needs to identify and conform with his or her peer group, and being 'different' (as teenagers with epilepsy will frequently perceive themselves to be) may result in social isolation (from their own, and opposite, sex) and reduced self-esteem and self-confidence. In addition, 'normal' adolescent behaviour that includes irregular patterns of sleeping and drinking may precipitate seizures. Conversely, the restriction of these 'normal' activities may result in the teenager feeling increasingly frustrated, angry with 'their' epilepsy and isolated, leading to anxiety, withdrawal and depression. These problems are compounded by the fact that the teenager is striving to become independent and attending clinic (GP or hospital), taking medication, relying on others and perceiving that their life is restricted in some way may, not surprisingly, have a detrimental effect on attempts to achieve this independence. The response of the family is clearly important in influencing how teenagers perceive their epilepsy and their attempts to gain independence. It is important that all aspects of epilepsy should be discussed openly within the family. It must also be recognized and understood that parental over-protectiveness is common (almost to the point of being expected) and that this over-protectiveness may result in either social isolation of the teenager (resulting in social and emotional ineptness) or frustration, anger and rebelliousness leading to antisocial, and even criminal, behaviour.

Teenagers may adopt a number of strategies in attempting to cope with the condition:

- Denial that they have epilepsy (including taking part, often to excess, in **all** normal adolescent behaviour, and non-compliance with both antiepileptic medication and clinic visits)

- Dissociation from the management of 'their' epilepsy, putting all the responsibility onto others and possibly blaming all their problems (e.g. poor results in examinations, inability to drive or the inability to secure a job or girlfriend/boyfriend) on 'my epilepsy'

Most young people find it uncomfortable and unacceptable to continue attending a paediatric clinic. The other most commonly offered alternatives are either to be discharged back to their GP or to be referred on to an adult physician (or, rarely, neurologist), who may not have an interest in epilepsy; these options are also frequently unsatisfactory. One approach would be a specific teenager clinic, which would fulfil many roles:[117,123]

1. To provide a further (and final) 'screen' to confirm (or refute) the diagnosis of epilepsy and corroborate (or correctly identify) the specific epilepsy syndrome

2. To ensure that the most appropriate drug is prescribed and, if possible, when and how the drug could be withdrawn

3. To address the specific social and psychological issues and concerns that are prevalent at this age

4. To provide a smooth hand-over of specialist care, from paediatric to adult services

5. To provide relevant and accurate information on career choice and restrictions, use (and abuse) of alcohol and driving licence regulations (see page 142)

The staffing of the teenager epilepsy clinic is also important and should certainly include a nurse specialist in epilepsy (who has a particular interest and skill in talking to young people and who is also able to visit the teenager at home or at college) as well as appropriately trained medical staff.[117] The nurse is often seen as being more approachable than a doctor and, particularly for young women, may be a more appropriate person to discuss more sensitive issues such as sex, contraception and pregnancy. However, it must be emphasized that satisfactorily addressing the psychosocial complications of epilepsy in teenagers may fall outside the expertise of both the neurologists (paediatric/adult) and nurse specialist and requires advice and support from clinical psychologists and psychiatrists – as well as specific career advice.

Information: teenagers generally prefer to be given facts and information rather than advice and recommendations. By giving them the facts and the relevant information, they can make the appropriate decisions, which is so important for their independence and self-empowerment. The information given to teenagers should be written or available on a DVD/CD – as well as orally and in a format that is relevant and intelligible. Examples of well-written teenager or young adult-friendly booklets include *Independence* (available from the authors) and *Epilepsy and the Young Adult* (available from Epilepsy Bereaved or EYA at 13 Crondace Road, London SW6 4BB).

Investigation of epilepsy

8

The reasons and aims of investigation in epilepsy are to classify the epilepsy syndrome, identify any obvious aetiology that might influence management (e.g. demonstration of a tumour) and facilitate discussion about prognosis (e.g. identification of a cerebral malformation) and recurrence/genetic risks (e.g. detection of a genetic syndrome or chromosomal abnormality).

As much clinical information as possible should be given when requesting an EEG or neuroimaging, including identifying any known or suspected provoking or triggering and relieving factors to the seizures. It is obviously important to state whether the child has any neurological deficit or asymmetry (e.g. hemiparesis, visual impairment or a ventriculo-peritoneal shunt in situ), and, when requesting neuroimaging, to also state whether an EEG had demonstrated any obvious focal abnormality or asymmetry. This information will enable the EEG and radiology departments to undertake the most relevant and appropriate investigations and it will also facilitate more clinically orientated neurophysiological and neuroradiological reports.

The investigation of children with epilepsy falls largely into three areas:

- Electroencephalography

  - routine; waking and sleep (natural, in preference to drug-induced sleep)

  - ambulatory

  - telemetry (simultaneous video-recording)

  - invasive or 'depth' electrode EEG (used rarely in children)

- Neuroimaging

  - computed tomography (CT)

  - magnetic resonance imaging (MRI) – which may be structural or functional

  - single photon emission computed tomography (SPECT)

  - positron emission tomography (PET)

- 'Other'

  - haematological; metabolic; molecular genetics; histological analysis (e.g. skin, muscle)

The role of the EEG[124,125]

The EEG is a frequently abused and misinterpreted investigation, primarily as it is considered to be a 'diagnostic' test for epilepsy, but also because of the normal maturational changes that develop with age, which are frequently reported as being abnormal or 'epileptiform'. It is also important to understand that a 'routine', outpatient EEG is recorded for only 25–30 minutes in the vast majority of EEG and neurophysiology departments. In addition, spontaneous clinical seizures are very unlikely to occur in the artificial setting of an EEG department.

However, the EEG is of value:

(a) As an aid to the clinical diagnosis of epilepsy: a single interictal EEG may, rarely, 'capture' a clinical seizure, even in the EEG department (e.g. typical absence or myoclonic seizure), but more commonly an interictal EEG is normal. Up to 50% of children with epilepsy will have a normal EEG. Repeated recordings, often sleep-deprived or undertaken during sleep, will reduce this number, and increase the identification of epileptiform activity. In contrast, 10–15% of the 'normal' paediatric population may show non-specific abnormalities and approximately 1–2% will show specific (spikes or sharp waves) epileptiform features without a history of clinical seizures. Thus, a routine interictal EEG can rarely, if ever, prove or disprove a diagnosis of epilepsy. Ambulatory EEG, or, more importantly, telemetry with the simultaneous video-recording of clinical events may be necessary in some children, particularly for nocturnal seizures, or to clarify whether frequent (usually daily) paroxysmal episodes are epileptiform or non-epileptic in origin.

(b) For the classification of epilepsy: the interictal and particularly the ictal EEG is useful in classifying the specific epilepsy syndrome, and in differentiating between primary and secondarily generalized seizures. A final clinical situation in which the EEG may in fact 'diagnose' as well as classify a seizure is non-convulsive status – either absence (spike-wave) or complex partial status. Both of these phenomena may be very difficult to recognize clinically, particularly in children with pre-existing learning or behavioural problems, or both.

(c) For the identification of a structural brain lesion or neurodegenerative disorder: focal abnormalities (characteristically a slow wave, but also a sharp wave or spike) may indicate the presence of an underlying structural lesion, including a tumour. This is far more commonly seen in adults, but may occur in children.[126] An asymmetric 'following response' during intermittent photic stimulation is also suggestive of an occipital lesion (the 'following response' absent or attenuated on the side of the lesion), particularly in older children and teenagers. The EEG may also demonstrate features suggesting a number of progressive neurodegenerative disorders, of which epileptic seizures are simply one manifestation, for example:

> - Large-amplitude spike and/or spike–slow-wave discharges coinciding with single flashes (1/second) on intermittent photic stimulation – late infantile neuronal ceroid lipofuscinosis ('Batten's disease')
> - Periodic high-amplitude sharp and slow-wave complexes (particularly during hyperventilation) repeated every 4–12 seconds – subacute sclerosing panencephalitis (SSPE)
> - Periodic lateralizing epileptiform discharges (PLEDS) – herpes simplex encephalitis; Alper's disease (progressive neuronal degeneration of childhood, with or without liver disease)
> - Others, including Angelman and Rett syndromes

(d) For monitoring response to treatment: this is rarely necessary, other than in typical absence epilepsy, as clinical absences may be unnoticed by parents/teachers, in non-convulsive status epilepticus and in West's syndrome, as the persistence or resolution of hypsarrhythmia is usually closely correlated with control of the spasms and, importantly, developmental prognosis.

(e) In the pre-surgical evaluation of epilepsy: in most situations, routine, surface EEG recordings with or without simultaneous video recording (video-EEG telemetry) will provide adequate information regarding the site of the obvious epileptogenic focus – or foci, particularly if MRI demonstrates a focal abnormality. However, where routine, surface EEG has not demonstrated a clear focus, invasive or 'depth' EEG recordings may be required using sphenoidal or foramen ovale-sited electrodes. Finally, where an epileptogenic focus appears to be sited close to an eloquent or functionally important area (sensory / motor cortex), brain surface recordings may be necessary – electrocorticography – using 'grids' or 'mats' of electrodes placed directly on the cortical surface.

Neuroimaging

Scanning the brains of all children with epilepsy is unnecessary. The indications include attempting to identify a cause for the seizures and occasionally for 'reassurance' (e.g. where other family members have had a brain tumour or arterio-venous malformation or when families really cannot accept a diagnosis of epilepsy and 'move on' without first knowing that a brain scan is 'normal').

- In children, brain tumours will be responsible for only 1–2% of all seizures and 4–6% of partial seizures
- In children who have an initial normal scan, later scans may reveal a slow-growing tumour only after months or years
- CT is an appropriate initial scanning technique for the exclusion of a brain tumour
- CT is less sensitive than MRI in detecting very small lesions, particularly within the temporal lobes, and in demonstrating subtle areas of dysgenesis and areas of abnormal grey matter (heterotopias) due to defective neuronal migration.[127] CT involves radiation, unlike MRI, and therefore MRI is generally preferable, particularly if repeat and serial neuroimaging is likely to be required
- CT more readily demonstrates intracranial calcification
- CT is (currently) more available and easier to perform; children undergoing MRI more frequently require a general anaesthetic, and MRI is more difficult to interpret
- MRI is the preferred imaging technique for children with complex partial seizures and infantile spasms

The following groups of children with epilepsy require a brain scan:

1. Children who have a neurological deficit/asymmetry (e.g. hemiparesis)
2. Children who have evidence of a neurocutaneous syndrome
3. Children with evidence of developmental regression
4. Children with simple partial seizures

5. Children with complex partial seizures (particularly if the seizures have clear frontal or temporal lobe features)
6. Children with infantile spasms or myoclonic seizures presenting in the first year of life
7. Children with persisting unclassifiable seizures
8. Children whose seizures relapse for no obvious reason following initial good control
9. Children under the age of 12 months who present with two or more complicated (particularly if focal or unilateral), 'febrile' seizure

It is equally important to recognize that certain children do not routinely require a brain scan:

1. Children with a primary (idiopathic) generalized epilepsy
2. Children with benign partial epilepsy with either centro-temporal or occipital spikes
3. Children with simple febrile seizures
4. A focal discharge on the EEG does not, in isolation, justify a brain scan

It has been recommended that brain imaging (with MRI) be undertaken in all children who present with a first seizure who do not have an idiopathic form of epilepsy.[128] This approach is neither rational nor practicable:

- A single seizure, even if epileptic in origin, does not diagnose epilepsy
- It may be very difficult, if not impossible, to determine whether, after a first epileptic seizure, the nature of the seizure is idiopathic or symptomatic

- It would be an inappropriate use of resources – particularly because many of these children would require either sedation or a general anaesthetic to achieve a successful scan – and sedation or general anaesthesia are not without risks, even though these risks may be small

- The positive yield of identifying an abnormality that would then require intervention (after only a single seizure) is likely to be very low.

There is no indication for undertaking a plain skull radiograph in children with epilepsy, and the use of cranial ultrasonography is limited to the neonatal period, primarily as an initial 'screening' investigation to document periventricular and intracerebral haemorrhage and to reveal any gross cerebral malformation.

Functional brain imaging is becoming increasingly available and useful, particularly in pre-surgical evaluation programmes.[129] Positron emission tomography (PET) scanning demonstrates hypometabolism in epileptic foci interictally, and is a sensitive and reliable indicator of the site of epileptogenic lesions. However, PET is an expensive technique that is available in only a few centres other than in the USA and is of limited use during a seizure. Single photon emission computed tomography (SPECT) is easier to interpret and cheaper, and shows both *hypoperfusion* in epileptic foci interictally, and *hyperperfusion* ictally and post-ictally (from 2–5 hours after a seizure). Functional MRI (fMRI) is rapidly evolving and is likely to be of greater practical use and may replace SPECT in the pre-

surgical evaluation of patients for epilepsy surgery.

The International League Against Epilepsy (ILAE) has published guidelines[130] for the neuroimaging of patients (including children) with epilepsy; as anticipated, MRI is considered to be the preferred modality, when available and providing there are no obvious medical contraindications (e.g. if the child has a cardiac pacemaker). These guidelines may be revised in the future with further advances in imaging techniques, including magneto-electroencephalography (MEEG) and functional MRI.

Finally, the combination of a good clinical history, adequate routine surface (scalp) EEG recording, high-resolution MRI and occasionally SPECT scanning has largely obviated the need for frequent invasive, depth EEG recording.

Other investigations

The type and extent of 'other' investigations that may be undertaken in children with epilepsy clearly depend on the specific clinical situation and the underlying diagnosis being considered. This is usually most relevant for the myoclonic epilepsies, and neurodegenerative (i.e. regressive) disorders that have epilepsy as a feature.

Some specific examples of syndromes
having epilepsy as a feature:

- *Mitochondrial cytopathy (MERFF and MELAS) – DNA analysis, muscle biopsy (to measure the activity of the respiratory chain enzymes)*

- *Neuronal ceroid lipofuscinoses (particularly late infantile and juvenile Batten's disease) – blood analysis (enzyme deficiency, DNA mutation), skin or rectal biopsy*

- *Other storage disorders – white blood cell (lysosomal) enzyme assay*

- *SSPE – serum and CSF measles antibodies*

- *Angelman syndrome – DNA analysis (microdeletion on chromosome 15)*

- *Rett syndrome – DNA analysis (MECP2 deletion on chromosome Xq28)*

- *Juvenile Huntington's disease – DNA analysis (abnormal trinucleotide repeats)*

See pages 74–77 for metabolic
investigations in epilepsy.

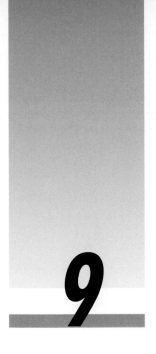

Drug treatment of epilepsy

There are a number of decisions that must be taken regarding the use of antiepileptic drugs (AEDs):

- *When to start a drug?*
- *Which drug and in what dose?*
- *When to change the drug?*
- *When to add a second drug (and which one)?*
- *When to seek a specialist opinion?*
- *When to stop the drug?*
- *When to measure blood levels of the drug?*
- *When to consider epilepsy surgery?*

When to start a drug?[131,132]

Most clinicians would not recommend starting treatment after a single brief generalized tonic–clonic seizure, but would after a cluster of seizures. Similarly, a child with severe physical and learning difficulties with infrequent myoclonic or brief partial seizures may not require an AED, in contrast to a child attending a normal school who experiences frequent generalized tonic–clonic seizures on waking. There are two main reasons why clinicians – and sometimes parents – are keen to start medication after one or only two seizures. Firstly, there has been the theoretical concern that one seizure may lead to a second and a second to a third and eventually to a state of chronic epilepsy that may be more difficult to treat. This process is termed 'kindling', where one seizure – which may be clinically or only electroencephalographically evident – 'begets another seizure' and so on; the evidence for this is primarily derived from rat data and has not been convincingly demonstrated in humans. Nevertheless, some clinicians still believe that early treatment after just one or two seizures may prevent the risk of the development of chronic and drug-resistant epilepsy. Recent data would suggest that this is most unlikely, providing the number of tonic–clonic seizures is 10 or less.[133,134] Secondly, is the concern that there may be an increased risk of injuries with further seizures and therefore early treatment may reduce this risk. Again, recent evidence has suggested that this is unlikely[135] and in fact physical injuries are probably more likely to occur in patients already diagnosed with epilepsy and receiving antiepileptic medication.[136]

Preliminary data from the national, Medical Research Council-sponsored, randomized study of epilepsy and single seizures (the 'MESS' Study) have suggested that seizure freedom after two years was almost identical (68%) for those patients randomized to early treatment with an AED (after one or two seizures) and those randomized to delayed treatment (after more than two seizures). Unfortunately, of the 1440 patients in this study, only 50 were aged less than five

years and only 440 were aged less than 19 years. This study also showed that for all 1440 patients, treatment with neither carbamazepine nor sodium valproate appeared to affect the prognosis of epilepsy at two years after diagnosis. (The results of this study are likely to be published in early 2004.)

Once an AED is started, the objective is to achieve (complete) seizure control without unacceptable side-effects and using the most appropriate formulation that can be taken by the child.

Which drug and in what dose?

It is the identification of the syndrome or (if no specific syndrome can be determined) the seizure type and safety profile of the drug that determine the choice of anticonvulsant. Whichever drug is chosen should be introduced gradually to avoid any dose-related side-effects, and increased slowly to its target maintenance dose based on the child's body weight and recommended guidelines. The dose of this drug should be increased to the maximally tolerated level before either adding a second drug (if the first drug has had a partial effect) or substituting another drug (if the first drug was completely ineffective).

The currently recommended first-line drugs in treating the majority of childhood epilepsies are sodium valproate (VPA) for generalized epilepsies and syndromes and carbamazepine (CBZ) for partial (focal) seizures/epilepsy syndromes. A previous randomized clinical trial (RCT) showed that VPA and CBZ were equally effective in both primary generalized tonic–clonic seizures and partial seizures with, or without, secondary generalization.[137] However, despite this evidence, it is the experience of many (including the authors) that sodium valproate is not particularly effective in treating partial seizures. For this reason the authors rarely use sodium valproate to treat partial (focal) seizures and epilepsies. Although ethosuximide may be effective for typical absences, it does not suppress tonic–clonic seizures, which may develop in 15–20% of children with childhood or juvenile-onset typical absence epilepsy. Ethosuximide may occasionally be of use in treating myoclonic seizures. Carbamazepine is effective in treating generalized tonic–clonic seizures, but exacerbates myoclonic and typical absence seizures and should therefore be avoided in juvenile myoclonic epilepsy and childhood-onset absence epilepsy. By the end of 2003, the National Institute for Clinical Excellence (NICE) will have published its report on the role and cost-effectiveness of the new AEDs compared with the older drugs (VPA and CBZ) in children and adults.

The only other syndrome/seizure type for which VPA and CBZ are not drugs of first choice is West's syndrome, which is characterized by infantile spasms. In the UK and Europe, vigabatrin is often the preferred drug.[138] In contrast to the USA, where adrenocorticotrophic hormone (ACTH) is the drug of choice,[139] in Japan the initial drug of choice in treating infantile spasms is pyridoxine (vitamin B6), for which it is reported that up to 10–15% of infants will respond (although this does not apparently imply that these infants have pyridoxine dependency, but simply that pyridoxine may occasionally be effective in treating some cases of infantile spasms). The mechanism of action of ACTH is unclear (although numerous hypotheses have been speculated), it has to be given by intramuscular injection (which is painful), and it is frequently associated with severe, and even fatal, side-effects. Prednisolone or hydrocortisone, commonly used alternative, oral steroids to ACTH/tetracosactrin, generally have both fewer and less serious side-effects. Vigabatrin is likely to suppress spasms in approximately 60% of patients, and prednisolone or ACTH in 65–70% of patients, depending upon the cause. Vigabatrin is particularly effective in treating infantile spasms caused by tuberous sclerosis.

Although vigabatrin has been linked with the development of symptomatic (and far more commonly asymptomatic), peripheral visual field constriction (possibly in up to 35–40% of adults treated with the drug), this should not preclude using vigabatrin as the initial first-choice drug in treating infantile spasms.[140] Current evidence suggests that early visual field constriction is seen after a minimum of six months' exposure to the drug and typically much longer

(2–3 years). The precise incidence of visual field constriction in children is not known, nor whether the visual field defect is reversible. If spasms show no reduction after 10 days of the maximum dose of vigabatrin (100–120 mg/kg/day), then it is very unlikely that this drug will be effective and it should be withdrawn and replaced with another drug (e.g. nitrazepam, prednisolone, pyridoxine, topiramate or sodium valproate).

Phenytoin and phenobarbitone must no longer be used as first-line maintenance drugs because of their relatively unsatisfactory side-effects, particularly on cognitive performance and behaviour and, with phenytoin, the cosmetic side-effects of gingival hyperplasia and hirsutism. These drugs should be considered for oral therapy only when other drugs have failed, and where seizure control is the over-riding – if not the only – priority.

When to change a drug or add a second drug?

If unacceptable side-effects develop or if control has been sub-optimal with the first drug then the child will require either a different AED (substitute drug) or an additional drug ('polytherapy'). The choice of the second drug is based on the same criteria as for the first drug – namely, seizure type or syndrome and safety profile. A single drug (monotherapy) will achieve total seizure control in 65–70% of children. Two drugs in combination will result in further significant (even complete) control in an additional 5–10% of children. Three drugs rarely (if ever) result in any additional control, and frequently cause more side-effects – and should therefore be avoided in most children and situations. First-, second- and third-choice drugs are shown in *Table 11*. Certain combinations of drugs must be used with caution *(Table 12)*.

Table 11
Drugs of first, second and third choice in the treatment of seizure types (largely reflecting current evidence and the authors' experience).

	First	Second	Third
Generalized			
Tonic–clonic	sodium valproate, lamotrigine	carbamazepine, topiramate	phenytoin
Myoclonic	sodium valproate	lamotrigine	ethosuximide, clonazepam, phenobarbitone
Tonic	sodium valproate	topiramate, lamotrigine, carbamazepine	clobazam, phenobarbitone
Atonic	sodium valproate	lamotrigine, topiramate	carbamazepine, clobazam, phenobarbitone
Absence	sodium valproate, ethosuximide	lamotrigine*	clobazam topiramate
Partial			
(simple/complex)†	carbamazepine	topiramate, gabapentin, clobazam,	lamotrigine, vigabatrin, phenytoin
Infantile spasms	vigabatrin§	nitrazepam, prednisolone	topiramate, ACTH‡, pyridoxine

* Recent evidence suggests that lamotrigine may be effective in treating typical absence seizures
† With, or without, secondary generalization
§ Vigabatrin is generally regarded (within the UK and Europe) as the drug of first choice, it may be effective in suppressing all spasms in 50–60% of children and the drug appears to work within 5–7 days of starting treatment; if the drug has not been effective after 10 days then it will not then be effective and should be replaced with another drug
‡ ACTH is not currently available in the UK; a synthetic 'equivalent' – tetracosactrin – is usually given in its place (by intramuscular injection)

(Levetiracetam is the newest AED; as of October 2003, it does not have a licence for use in children aged under 16 years. However, early evidence suggests that as well as being effective in treating partial seizures, either with or without secondary generalization, the drug may also be effective in some primary generalized seizures. The drug does not appear to interact with other AEDs or with oral contraceptives.)

Table 12
Drug combinations that should be avoided or used with caution.

- Carbamazepine and valproate (increased carbamazepine toxicity)
- Carbamazepine and lamotrigine (possible increased carbamazepine toxicity)
- Valproate and phenytoin (loss of efficacy of valproate)
- Ethosuximide and phenytoin (increased phenytoin toxicity)
- Valproate and lamotrigine (potentially a very effective combination in treating primary generalized seizures but caution needed because of the risk of a severe rash, tremor, drowsiness and headache)

When to seek a specialist opinion?

If, after 4–6 months' treatment, or less if the child's seizures are frequent, with one, or at most two, drugs in maximally tolerated doses, seizure control remains difficult, unacceptable or both, then advice should be sought from a specialist with an interest in epilepsy – a paediatric neurologist. This is important for the following reasons:

- An increased knowledge and understanding of all the epilepsy syndromes and the role and potential problems in using the new antiepileptic drugs
- An increased awareness of potential underlying and progressive neurodegenerative conditions
- Access to more detailed investigations, and how to use them appropriately
- Access to a centre for epilepsy surgery
- Improved access to neuropsychology, psychiatry and counselling – should this be necessary

When to stop the drug?[141,142]

This again depends largely on the epilepsy syndrome, but also the wishes of the child/family and the social/educational situation. Certain syndromes are associated with a high rate of relapse if the drug is withdrawn (e.g. juvenile myoclonic epilepsy), others with a low risk (e.g. childhood-onset absence epilepsy and benign partial epilepsy with rolandic spikes). The overall risk of relapse is approximately 20–25% in children. Factors known to influence the risk of relapse include:

- Duration of remission (long duration – lower risk)
- Time taken to achieve remission (shorter time – lower risk)
- Generalized tonic–clonic seizures (presence – higher risk)
- Myoclonic seizures (presence – higher risk)
- Spikes or slow-wave activity on EEG (presence – higher risk)

Most clinicians would usually suggest attempted withdrawal of an AED after a seizure-free period of 2–3 years; this is essentially an arbitrary figure. Prospective data have shown that in children who became seizure-free within a few months after receiving their first AED, the risk of seizure recurrence was no different when the drug was withdrawn after six months of seizure freedom (51% seizure-free), compared with 12 months of seizure freedom (52% seizure-free).[143] Predictive factors for relapse after withdrawal of medication included partial seizures, seizure onset (of any type) occurring after 12 years of age and an identified cause for the epilepsy. In the absence of these factors it may therefore be worth considering withdrawal of antiepileptic medication after 12 months of seizure freedom, rather than the currently recommended – but arbitrary – period of 24 months. Evidence also suggests that after an initial failed attempt at drug withdrawal, firstly, seizure-control is likely to be regained and secondly a subsequent attempt at withdrawing medication may still be successful.[144,145]

Many recommend repeating an EEG before discontinuing a drug, although the decision to withdraw should be based primarily on clinical rather than EEG criteria.[146] The identification of spike and slow-wave activity on the EEG before withdrawing an AED will increase the risk of that child/teenager experiencing seizures either during or after withdrawal, but this does not mean that further seizures will definitely occur. Similarly, a 'normal' EEG prior to withdrawal cannot guarantee that there will be no seizure recurrence. Obviously, the implications of seizure recurrence following withdrawal and discontinuation of an AED are different for children and older teenagers/young adults, particularly if the latter already have driving licences/employment. In the authors'

experience most children (and their parents) and teenagers do decide to try to discontinue medication at least once; not infrequently this is undertaken without their parent's (or the doctor's) knowledge.

AEDs must be discontinued gradually to prevent withdrawal seizures, particularly with phenobarbitone or the benzodiazepines; sudden discontinuation may also precipitate convulsive status epilepticus (and this is one of the most common causes of status in the teenager and young adult with epilepsy). A withdrawal period of 6–8 weeks (occasionally 3 months for benzodiazepines) is appropriate for most drugs; one study showed no difference between 6 weeks and 9 months.[147] Rarely, seizure control may be difficult to regain after drug withdrawal, following an initial period of good control.

When to measure a blood level?[148]

This is undertaken far too frequently, and should be limited to the following situations:

- *Where major non-compliance is suspected*
- *When a child with epilepsy presents in convulsive/non-convulsive status epilepticus (the levels may be too low or, rarely, too high)*
- *When the child has learning or communication difficulties and is unable to describe symptoms of toxicity*
- *Children taking phenytoin (particularly as part of 'polytherapy')*

The lower and upper limits of the blood levels of most AEDs are arbitrarily defined and have no clear clinical correlation. Most children with epilepsy will be controlled with blood levels below the stated 'therapeutic ranges'. Not infrequently, blood level monitoring can lead to patients who are adequately controlled, with low blood levels, having their doses needlessly increased (with extra risk of side-effects), and to patients who need relatively high blood levels of an AED for adequate seizure control (and who tolerate such high levels with no side-effects), having doses needlessly reduced, thereby increasing the risk of experiencing further seizures. Full blood counts, serum electrolytes and liver function tests should also not be undertaken routinely, but only when clinically indicated.

When to consider surgery?

Any patient with partial seizures refractory to optimal doses of conventional AEDs and whose prognosis for spontaneous seizure remission is poor should be considered for surgical treatment. It is important that surgery is not delayed excessively; most specialists would recommend a period of no longer than 2 years (of poor seizure control) using three or four antiepileptic drugs (sequentially and not in combination) in maximally tolerated doses, before discussing possible surgery, but this period could, and probably should, be much shorter in specific situations, particularly if an abnormality has been demonstrated on neuroimaging.

Communication

At the start of treatment parents (and where appropriate, the child) must be informed about:

- The seizure type and whenever possible the specific epilepsy/epilepsy syndrome
- The likely prognosis
- The aims and duration of treatment
- The likely and unlikely side-effects of the AED
- The importance of compliance – taking medication regularly and as prescribed

Ideally this information should be provided in both verbal and written form.[149]

Changes in drugs or their dosages must also be communicated to the general practitioner, the relevant school doctor (clinical medical officer) and the school nurse. The importance of good communication cannot be overemphasized, particularly between the hospital and the community, including the school. This can be greatly improved through the use of 'nurse specialists' or 'liaison nurses' in paediatric epilepsy.

Management of epilepsy associated with other cerebral disorders

This follows the same principles as in the management of isolated epilepsy. Partial seizures, with or without secondary generalization, are the most common seizure type in children with structural brain lesions but generalized seizures are also common. Epilepsy occurring in association with other cerebral disorders is generally more difficult to control and, especially in children with severe learning difficulties, poses additional management problems:

- *Seizure control is usually incomplete; so in many cases 'polytherapy' may be necessary – with all the potential problems of using two AEDs simultaneously*

- *Compliance with antiepileptic medication*

- *Assessment of seizure control*

- *Assessment of side-effects of drugs (particularly cognitive dysfunction, drowsiness, ataxia)*

- *Occurrence and recognition of pseudo-epileptic seizures (non-epileptic seizures) and, importantly, non-convulsive status epilepticus*

- *There is an increased risk of dying prematurely in this specific group of patients – including as a result of a tonic–clonic seizure itself, the underlying cause of epilepsy and 'SUDEP'* [4–6,11,12]

Complex partial (a form of non-convulsive) status epilepticus is not that uncommon in children who have epilepsy and learning /behaviour difficulties and usually requires an EEG to confirm (or exclude) the diagnosis (this is discussed in more detail in Chapter 12 on Status epilepticus).

The adverse effects of AEDs may impair the overall functioning of children who have significant physical and intellectual disabilities, even though seizure control is improved. In some children periods without an anticonvulsant (AED) may be

appropriate. In children with refractory epilepsy whose seizures have persisted despite having received most of the available AEDs, parents often ask if all the drugs can be stopped. They want to know if their child could be more alert and have less behavioural problems (but with no worsening of seizure control), if their child were receiving no medication. This is a reasonable request but parents need to be forewarned that there is an increased risk that their child may have more major seizures, including convulsive status epilepticus, even if the antiepileptic medication is gradually withdrawn.

The issue of side-effects is clearly very important and is of perennial concern to parents of children with epilepsy – to the point where antiepileptic medication may be declined if their child's seizures occur only during sleep, are brief (partial or myoclonic) or infrequent (months or even years apart). Another reason for refusing medication may reflect what they might have heard from often well-meaning family members or friends, or found on the internet about these drugs, particularly if this included reading the full data sheet on the drug (as published by the drug company), personal anecdotes or families' experiences from around the world. It is clear from the authors' experience that these fears and perceptions may be difficult to dispel. However, it is also clear that children vary considerably in their response to AEDs, not just in terms of seizure control but also (and more frequently) in terms of tolerability; some children are able to tolerate very high doses of a drug whilst others of the same age and sex can barely tolerate any dose. It is certainly possible that there may be a genetic predisposition to the development of adverse side-effects with AEDs, as a number of the enzymes that are involved in their metabolism are associated with genetic polymorphisms. These adverse drug reactions or side-effects may be mild (e.g. drowsiness, tremor, behaviour changes) or severe (e.g. hepatitis, pancreatitis, Stevens–Johnson syndrome, bone marrow suppression). This clearly deserves further evaluation and is potentially an exciting area of pharmacological – and genetic (i.e. pharmacogenomic) – research within epilepsy. Clinically, it also emphasizes the need to:

- Use one drug in the lowest possible dose to achieve seizure control

- Use no more than two drugs simultaneously (if more than one drug is required)

- Listen to the family and carers when they describe their children's response to the antiepileptic medication that is prescribed

- Document (and report) all apparently genuine adverse side-effects or adverse drug reactions

When seizure control improves only temporarily following the introduction of an AED, then using drugs on a rotational basis at regular intervals might produce a more sustained period of seizure control – although this is somewhat theoretical and in the authors' experience is rarely successful.

Finally, but no less importantly, the presence of learning difficulties and/or behavioural problems does not necessarily preclude epilepsy surgery, whichever procedure is contemplated or being considered.

AEDs and their characteristics

Acetazolamide	
Trade name	*Diamox*
Mode of action	*Carbonic anhydrase inhibitor; 'anticonvulsant' mechanism of action unclear*
Indications	*Add-on (usually to carbamazepine) for simple and complex partial (including atypical absence) seizures*
Dose	
Children	*8–30 mg/kg per day (2–4 divided doses)*
Optimal range	*Not routinely measured*
Side-effects	
Dose-related	*Malaise, fatigue, headache, drowsiness, paraesthesia of face and limbs, metabolic acidosis, tinnitus*
Allergic	*Leucopenia, thrombocytopenia and aplastic anaemia, skin rash*
Chronic toxicity	*Electrolyte disturbance (hypokalaemia) and acidosis; renal calculi*

Carbamazepine

Trade name *Tegretol; Tegretol Retard*

Mode of action *Limits repetitive firing of Na⁺-dependent action potentials*

Mode of action *Limits repetitive firing of Na^+-dependent action potentials*

Indications *Drug of choice: simple and complex partial, and tonic–clonic seizures. May be effective in tonic seizures. Exacerbates myoclonic and typical absence seizures*

Dose

 Children *<1 yr – 100–200 mg; 1–5 yr – 200–400 mg; 5–10 yr – 400–600 mg; 10–15 yr – 0.6–1.0 g or commence on 5 mg/kg per day for 7–14 days and increase up to 10–20 mg/kg per day over the next 14–21 days. The sustained-release preparation (Tegretol Retard) may be useful in avoiding the dose-related side-effects*

 Optimal range *4–10 µg/ml (but little evidence to support this)*

Side-effects

 Dose-related *Dizziness, double vision, unsteadiness, nausea and vomiting. Exacerbates myoclonic and typical absence seizures, and polyspike/spike and wave on the EEG*

 Allergic *Rashes (2–5% of all patients), reduced white cell count*

 Chronic toxicity *Few known: absence of major effects on intellectual function and behaviour is major benefit*

Clobazam

Trade name *Frisium*

Mode of action *Allosteric enhancement of GABA-mediated inhibition*

Indications *Useful as adjunctive treatment for tonic–clonic, tonic/atonic, absence and partial seizures; used premenstrually, for seizure clusters (catamenial seizures) and also prophylactically to prevent seizures induced by stressful events (e.g. examinations, holidays, travel etc.)*

Dose

 Children *0.5–1.0 (maximum 2) mg/kg per day*

 Optimal range *Not routinely measured*

Side-effects

 Dose-related *Drowsiness; sedation; rarely irritability*

 Chronic toxicity *Tachyphylaxis and tolerance (less than with other benzodiazepines)*

Clonazepam

Trade name *Rivotril*

Mode of action *Allosteric enhancement of GABA-mediated inhibition*

Indications *Drug of choice: myoclonic seizures and hyperekplexia*
Effective in: myoclonus, absence
Occasional use: tonic–clonic and partial seizures (value greatly limited by development of tolerance)

Dose

 Children   <1 yr – 0.5–1.0 mg/day;
       1–5 yr – 1–3 mg/day; 6–12 yr
       – 3–6 mg/day or
       0.1–0.2 mg/kg per day, but
       commence on 0.02 mg/kg per
       day

 Optimal range   Not routinely measured

Side-effects

 Dose-related   Sedation and drowsiness;
       irritability

 IV   Inflammation of veins

Diazepam

Trade name   Valium; Diazemuls; Stesolid

Mode of action   Allosteric enhancement of GABA-
       mediated inhibition

Indications   Status epilepticus (currently drug
       of choice for non-intravenous use;
       lorazepam is the drug of choice for
       intravenous use)
       Very rarely used as maintenance
       in absence or myoclonus (role
       limited by development of
       tolerance); clonazepam and
       clobazam are the preferred
       maintenance oral benzodiazepines

Dose

 Children   0.4–0.5 mg/kg (intravenous or
       rectal administration)
       Little effect orally

 Optimal range   Not routinely measured

Side-effects
 Dose-related   Sedation; irritability

 Chronic toxicity   Habituation

Ethosuximide

Trade name   Zarontin; Emeside

Mode of action   ?Reduces low-threshold calcium
       current in thalamus
       ?Enhancement of non-GABA-
       mediated inhibition

Indications   Typical absences; myoclonus

Dose

 Children   <6 yr – 250 mg/day; >6 yr –
       0.5–1.0 g/day or
       20–40 mg/kg per day

 Optimal range   40–100 µg/ml

Side-effects

 Dose-related   Nausea, drowsiness, dizziness,
       unsteadiness, may exacerbate
       tonic–clonic seizures, chronic,
       daily headaches

 Allergic   Rashes; bone marrow suppression

Felbamate

Trade name   Not currently available in the UK

Mode of action   Uncertain; multiple mechanisms
       possibly including blockade of
       sodium channels, indirect NMDA
       receptor antagonism and possibly
       GABA potentiation

Indications   Currently, in the USA, one of the
       drugs indicated specifically for the
       Lennox–Gastaut syndrome. Also
       effective against partial and
       generalized seizures

Dose

 Children   15–40 mg/kg per day
       Although this drug has been
       withdrawn in the UK (1994)

owing to its association with aplastic anaemia, its use continues to slowly increase in the USA

Optimal range	Not yet established

Side-effects

Dose-related	Dose-related nausea, weight loss, insomnia, increases phenytoin but decreases carbamazepine levels; hepatitis
Allergic	Hepatoxicity (potentially fatal), aplastic anaemia (potentially fatal), skin rash
Chronic toxicity	Not yet known

Gabapentin

Trade name	Neurontin
Mode of action	Binds to a novel calcium channel receptor
Indications	Refractory partial or generalized tonic–clonic seizures (primary or secondary generalized)

Dose

Children	>12 yr – 300–2400 mg/day or 15–50 mg/kg per day (all ages)
Optimal range	Not yet established

Side-effects

Dose-related	Mild sedation, unsteadiness, behaviour changes
Allergic	None yet identified
Chronic toxicity	Not yet known

Lamotrigine

Trade name	Lamictal
Mode of action	Diminished release of excitatory amino acid (glutamate)
Indications	Refractory partial and generalized seizures; useful in the Lennox–Gastaut syndrome and for typical and atypical absence seizures. Useful in juvenile myoclonic epilepsy

Dose

Children	Maintenance dose: 1–4 mg/kg per day (with sodium valproate).* Maintenance dose: 2–15 mg/kg per day (without sodium valproate)
Optimal range	Not yet established

Side-effects

Dose-related	Mild sedation, blurred vision, ataxia, nausea and vomiting, headache, diplopia, tremor (particularly if already receiving sodium valproate)
Allergic	Rashes (2–4%; higher if drug introduced rapidly); hepatoxicity (rare)
Chronic toxicity	Not yet known

*When added to sodium valproate, lamotrigine must be introduced in a very low dose, and increased gradually. The commencing dose is 0.2–0.3 mg/kg per day, and the dose should be increased only every 2 weeks up to the initial target maintenance dose

Levetiracetam

Trade name	Keppra
Mode of action	Unknown; antiepileptogenic rather than antiseizure effect. No demonstratable effect on the GABA, benzodiazepine, or excitatory amino acid receptors. Possible selective stereospecific binding site in the brain
Indications	Add-on therapy for adults and children (>16 years of age) with refractory partial seizures with or without secondary generalization
Dose	
Children	Maintenance dose: 30–40 mg/kg per day given as a twice-daily regime. Starting dose is 5–10 mg/kg per day increasing every 2 weeks up to the maintenance dose
Optimal range	Not yet established
Side-effects	
Dose-related	Somnolence, asthenia and dizziness. Headache and mild gastro-intestinal symptoms are less common. No major interaction with other antiepileptic drugs or with oral contraceptives
Allergic	None known
Chronic toxicity	Not yet known

Oxcarbazepine

Trade name	Trileptal
Mode of action	Limits repetitive firing of Na^+-dependent action potentials (similar to carbamazepine)
Indications	Simple and complex partial seizures; primary and secondary generalized tonic–clonic seizures. Avoid in myoclonic and typical absence seizures
Dose	
Children	Starting dose of 5–10 mg/kg per day, increasing over 4–6 weeks to 30 mg/kg per day (a slightly higher-dose regime than with carbamazepine)
Optimal range	Not yet established ('target' blood level of 12–30 µg/ml for purposes of assessing compliance or toxicity)
Side-effects	
Dose-related	Reported to be less frequent than with carbamazepine. Fatigue, dizziness, double-vision, unsteadiness, nausea and vomiting. These reduced side-effects are due to the fact that oxcarbazepine, unlike carbamazepine, is not metabolized to an epoxide product. Exacerbates myoclonic and typical absence seizures
Allergic	Maculopapular rash in 5–10% of patients (worth considering if patients developed a rash with carbamazepine, as there appears to be only 25–33% cross-reactivity)

Chronic toxicity   *Reduced white cell count; hyponatraemia (more common than with carbamazepine but usually mild and of no clinical significance). Limited data suggest no major effects on psychological or cognitive function*

Phenobarbitone

Trade name   *Gardenal; Luminal; Prominal*

Mode of action   *Enhancement of GABA-mediated inhibition*

Indications   *One of the first-line, intravenous long-acting drugs in convulsive status epilepticus; also effective in tonic, clonic and partial seizures Occasional oral use: absence, myoclonus, tonic–clonic seizures*

Dose
   Children   *2–8 mg/kg per day given either once or twice daily. Rarely higher doses may be necessary (under 1 yr of age)*

   Optimal range   *15–35 µg/ml; both upper and lower limits modified by development of tolerance*

Side-effects
   Dose-related   *Drowsiness, unsteadiness, irritability*

   Allergic   *Rashes*

   Chronic toxicity   *Tolerance, habituation, withdrawal seizures. Adverse effects on intellectual function and behaviour*

Phenytoin

Trade name   *Epanutin*

Mode of action   *Inhibits sustained repetitive firing effects on Na⁺-dependent voltage channels*

Indications   *Treatment of generalized tonic–clonic and partial seizures not satisfactorily controlled by other drugs. Treatment of choice (as an i.v. infusion) for convulsive status epilepticus when a long-acting anticonvulsant is required (fosphenytoin may replace phenytoin in status epilepticus; see Chapter 12 on Status epilepticus)*

Dose
   Children   *3–8 mg/kg per day; neonates often require 15–20 mg/kg per day*

   Optimal range   *10–20 µg/ml; the non-linear relationship between dose and serum concentration necessitates blood-level monitoring*

Side-effects
   Dose-related   *Drowsiness, ataxia, slurred speech, occasionally abnormal movement disorders (choreiform; athetoid)*

   Allergic   *Rashes, swelling of lymph glands (pseudolymphoma), hepatitis*

   Chronic toxicity   *Gingival hypertrophy, acne, coarsening of facial features, hirsutism, folate deficiency, osteomalacia*

Primidone

Trade name	*Mysoline*
Mode of action	*As phenobarbitone*
Indications	*Occasional use: tonic–clonic and partial seizures; rarely used in children*

Dose

Children	*10–30 mg/kg in 2 or 3 doses*
Optimal range	*As phenobarbitone, to which it is metabolized*

Side-effects

Dose-related	*Drowsiness; unsteadiness; tolerated poorly on initiation, and a slow increase in dose advisable*
Allergic	*See phenobarbitone*
Chronic toxicity	*See phenobarbitone*

Sodium valproate

Trade name	*Epilim; Epilim Chrono*
Mode of action	*?Enhancement of GABA-mediated inhibition* *?Limits sustained repetitive firing of neurones* *?Reduces effects of excitatory amino acid (glutamate)*
Indications	*Drug of choice: idiopathic generalized epilepsies (including typical absences), myoclonic seizures and photosensitive epilepsy* *May occasionally be useful in partial seizures – but not as a drug of second or even third choice* *Occasionally effective in infantile spasms (high dose)*

Dose

Children	*20–60 mg/kg per day (usually 20–40 mg/kg per day; higher doses in infantile spasms)* *A modified-release version (Epilim Chrono) is available for once-daily administration*
Optimal range	*Uncertain: blood levels vary considerably during the day, and a single specimen is unreliable*

Side-effects

Dose-related	*Tremor, irritability, restlessness Occasionally confusion including encephalopathy; cognitive and behavioural difficulties may be more common than is currently believed/accepted*
Allergic	*Gastric intolerance, hepatotoxicity (mainly in children under the age of 3 years with myoclonic seizures, mental retardation and receiving multiple AEDs)*
Chronic toxicity	*Weight gain, alopecia, menstrual irregularities (mainly amenorrhoea) including polycystic ovaries and a reported association with the polycystic ovary syndrome*

Tiagabine

Trade name	Gabitril
Mode of action	Inhibits the neuronal and glial uptake of GABA after its release from postsynaptic GABA receptors (the drug therefore enhances GABA-mediated inhibition)
Indications	Add-on therapy for adults and children (>12 years of age) with refractory partial seizures with or without secondary generalization
Dose	
Children	Limited data available: maintenance dose: 30 mg/day given twice or three times a day. Starting dose is 5 mg/day increasing every one or two weeks (with increments of 5 mg/day) to the initial maximum dose of 30 mg/day
Optimal range	Not yet established
Side-effects	
Dose-related	Dizziness, fatigue, somnolence, tremor and difficulty concentrating, 'knee-buckling' when walking (usually in high doses); reported association with complex partial status epilepticus in some patients
Allergic	None known
Chronic toxicity	Not yet known; no reports of peripheral visual field constriction

Topiramate

Trade name	Topamax
Mode of action	Multiple: a) blocks voltage-activated sodium channels b) stimulates GABA-A receptors c) blocks glutamate receptors d) weak carbonic anhydrase inhibitor
Indications	Newly presenting or refractory partial or generalized tonic–clonic seizures (may be particularly effective for tonic and atonic seizures); Lennox Gastaut syndrome
Dose	
Children	2–10 (usually 5–6) mg/kg/day. The commencing dose is 0.5 mg/kg/day, given as a once-daily dose and increased gradually every two weeks, up to an initial maintenance dose of 5–6 mg/kg/day given as two divided doses
Optimal range	Not yet established; serum monitoring not usually required
Side-effects	
Dose-related	Anorexia and either no increase in weight or weight loss; sedation, fatiguability, impaired concentration, dizziness, behavioural changes
Allergic	None known
Chronic toxicity	Renal stones (predominantly reported in adults); decreased sweating. Adverse effects on cognitive function (some cognitive slowing) Depression and psychosis with aggression (rare)

Vigabatrin	
Trade name	Sabril
Mode of action	Enzyme-activated suicidal inhibitor of GABA-aminotransaminase therefore increasing GABA-mediated inhibition
Indications	Treatment of partial epilepsy not satisfactorily controlled by other drugs. One of the drugs of choice in infantile spasms (West's syndrome)
Dose	
Children	Infantile spasms: 50–120 mg/kg per day (in two divided doses), partial seizures: 40–80 mg/kg per day (in two divided doses), but only to a maximum of 3 g per day
Optimal range	Unrelated to known mode of action
Side-effects	Few; mild drowsiness, occasional behavioural changes (irritability, very rarely a reversible psychosis) May exacerbate myoclonic and typical absence seizures and polyspike/spike and wave on EEG
Chronic toxicity	Probably dose-related effect on peripheral visual fields (constriction of visual fields with temporal sparing); incidence in children unclear (?20–30%; 35–40% in adults) and possibly irreversible, but long-term data are not yet available

Drugs on the horizon

There are a number of AEDs that are currently being developed or undergoing clinical trials. These include drugs in:

- phase II and III clinical trials (to obtain initial efficacy and safety data, almost exclusively in adults to obtain an initial product licence)
- phase IV clinical trials (in an attempt to achieve new indications for an already licensed drug, such as for paediatric use or for use as monotherapy).

In addition some drugs with a product licence for use in epilepsy are already being prescribed in countries other than Great Britain.

Remacemide

This drug has been in the process of development for many years. Its mechanism of action is by non-competitive inhibition of N-methyl-D-aspartic acid (NMDA) receptors – a component of the most potent excitatory neurotransmitter system within the central nervous system. The drug may also act by blocking sodium channels. Clinical data are limited to its use in partial seizures in adults with some response but overall the drug appears to have a lower efficacy than carbamazepine. Simultaneous use of other AEDs may result in increased blood levels of carbamazepine and phenytoin. Dosing is either two, three or four times a day and the most common and dose-limiting side-effects include dizziness, fatigue and gastrointestinal disturbance (nausea, vomiting, dyspepsia). The role of remacemide in the future treatment of epilepsy is uncertain.

Stiripentol

This drug may be effective in myoclonic seizures with or without absences, and particularly in children with severe myoclonic epilepsy in infancy. There is potential interaction with other AEDs (specifically carbamazepine and sodium valproate) in view of its hepatic metabolism through the cytochrome P450 system. Drowsiness, hyperexcitability and aggression are the most commonly reported adverse side-effects. Limited data suggest a starting dose of 10 mg/kg/day increasing over four weeks up to a maximum of 40–50 mg/kg/day, using a twice-daily regime.

Sulthiame

This drug was introduced in the early 1960s and has remained popular in Germany and Europe but is rarely used in the UK and USA. Structurally related to sulphanilamide and acetazolamide, its anti-seizure mechanism of action is thought to be due to its weak carbonic anhydrase inhibitory effect, although there may be other mechanisms of action. It appears to be effective against partial and also myoclonic seizures (and myoclonic–astatic epilepsy), but rarely against tonic–clonic seizures. Side-effects include hyperpnoea and dyspnoea, which may necessitate discontinuation of the

drug. Additional adverse side-effects include distal paraesthesiae, poor co-ordination, somnolence and, rarely, psychosis. The drug has to be given at least twice, if not three times, daily. When given simultaneously with other AEDs, blood levels of phenytoin are increased, which may in part explain sulthiame's efficacy in partial seizures. The drug cannot currently be considered as a first-choice drug for any seizure type.

Zonisamide

This is a potentially broad-spectrum drug that is reported to be effective in a number of seizure types, including partial seizures with or without secondary generalization, myoclonic seizures and, in Japanese studies, 'refractory' infantile spasms. There are very few randomized clinical trial data. The drug is related to the sulphonamides; it is partially metabolized in the liver and its excretion is predominantly renal. It is poorly bound to plasma proteins and there appear to be no clinically significant interactions with most other AEDs. Its mechanism of action is multiple, including blockage of voltage-sensitive sodium channels, inhibition of voltage-dependent T-type calcium channels and facilitation of dopaminergic and serotoninergic neurotransmission, although it is unclear which is/are responsible for its anticonvulsant action. The drug also weakly inhibits carbonic anhydrase and may potentially protect neurones from free-radical damage. Adverse side-effects include somnolence, ataxia, anorexia and confusion. Renal stones have been reported from studies in the USA (approximately 2–3%) but not in Japan (approximately 0.2%). The starting dose in children is 1 mg/kg/day, increasing every two weeks up to a maximum of 4 mg/kg/day using a twice-daily regime. Currently the drug is available in capsule form only. Zonisamide may be licensed for adjunctive use in the UK in 2003/4 for adults with refractory partial epilepsy.

Pregabilin

This is related to gabapentin but is reported to be considerably more potent in early clinical trials in adults; paediatric studies will follow.

Others

Rufinamide and valrocemide... and still more currently 'over the horizon'!

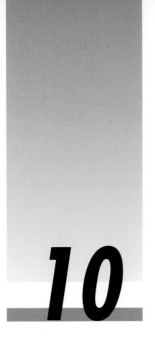

Surgical treatment of epilepsy

Surgical intervention is now recognized as a therapeutic option for many children with refractory seizures.[150,151] It is also clear that for many surgery is undertaken far too late, with social and educational implications. However, the surgical treatment of epilepsy, once undertaken, is irreversible. It is therefore crucial to ensure that, firstly, the child has epilepsy which is resistant to antiepileptic medication, and, secondly, that surgery is likely to either prevent or at least markedly reduce further seizures – and as a direct consequence, their quality of life.

For surgery to be effective the epileptogenic region (focus) must either be removed (resective surgery) or 'disconnected' from other non-epileptogenic cerebral tissue, thereby preventing or at least limiting a secondary generalized tonic–clonic seizure. Successful resective surgery depends upon the accurate localization of the focus, which is the primary objective of any pre-surgical evaluation.

The patient

Patients must fulfil a number of criteria before being considered for surgery:

> 1. Persisting intractable seizures despite maximally tolerated doses of antiepileptic drugs. (There is no generally agreed period of drug-resistant seizures before surgery is considered, although the figure of 2 years is often quoted, which for many patients is too long. The period of observation demonstrating medical intractability depends on the seizure type and frequency, epilepsy type and aetiology)
>
> 2. No realistic hope of a spontaneous remission of the epilepsy
>
> 3. Evidence of medical, social and educational disability due to the seizures, with the child's 'quality of life' likely to improve after surgery
>
> 4. Acceptable risk–benefit ratio for the proposed surgery
>
> 5. Diagnostic investigations point to a common (single) epileptogenic focus; (any discordant result(s) adversely affects the outcome of surgery, with regard to both seizure control and psychosocial functioning)

The pre-surgical evaluation[152]

This is clearly very important, differs between centres and is continually changing. Most evaluation programmes would include the following parameters:

> 1. Detailed clinical history and seizure pattern
>
> 2. Scalp EEG (background, interictal and ictal findings)
>
> 3. Video-EEG telemetry to record a number of the patient's typical seizures and identify a single focus – and (hopefully) exclude multiple foci responsible for the seizures
>
> 4. Neuroimaging (MRI is superior to CT and is essential prior to any surgery)

> 5. Neuropsychometry (including the intracarotid amytal or 'WADA' test. This test is rarely possible in children under 10 years of age. The information derived from the test is crucial in assessing not only the dominant hemisphere for memory and speech, but also whether the temporal lobe contralateral to that of proposed surgical resection could sustain memory independently)

If the above tests are concordant, identifying a single focus and a visible structural lesion (e.g. focal cortical dysplasia, mesial temporal sclerosis, a DNET, a single epileptogenic tuber in tuberous sclerosis or the angiomatous malformation in Sturge–Weber syndrome) then no further investigations are usually required. However, if the scalp EEG shows no clear lateralization or the MRI demonstrates no obvious lesion (or both) then further, more invasive studies may be required, including:

> • More detailed video-EEG monitoring – with scalp or more likely foramen ovale/sphenoidal EEG recording
>
> • Interictal but more importantly ictal SPECT (SPECT is more readily available and cheaper than PET, and ictal events cannot be recorded easily with PET)
>
> • Interictal SPECT is of limited use without ictal SPECT in trying to identify an obvious focus
>
> • Intracranial/subdural electrode recording (this method of recording the EEG is particularly invasive, and is usually reserved for differentiating between temporal and extratemporal foci)

The advent of more advanced structural but particularly functional (SPECT and, most recently, MRI) neuroimaging has obviated the need for routine depth electrode recording in most patients undergoing surgical evaluation. However, where resective surgery is being considered in 'eloquent' areas of the brain, close to important functional areas (e.g. the motor cortex), then pre-operative and/or intra-operative cortical recordings using a series of electrodes in either a 'grid' or 'map' may be required; this is called electrocorticography. These electrodes may be used to not only record but also stimulate the area of motor cortex in and around the site of possible resection to try and determine the precise localization of motor function – and thus what function might possibly be lost or impaired – and therefore guide the neurosurgeon as to the lines of a 'safe' resection.

The procedure

The commonly performed procedures are either resective (temporal and extratemporal lobe, multilobar or hemispherectomy) or functional (stereotactic or disconnective). Resective surgery aims to be curative, disconnective surgery more palliative. The rationale and indications for these different surgical techniques are shown in **Table 13**.

Surgery must be undertaken in a recognized, national centre with comprehensive pre- and post-surgical (including psychological) evaluation and support facilities.

The outcome (in terms of seizure control)[153,154]

The limited outcome data for epilepsy surgery in children are similar to those in adults. Seizure freedom can be expected in approximately:

- *70–75% undergoing temporal lobe resections*
- *30–40% undergoing extratemporal (usually frontal) lobe resections (this relatively poor outcome reflects an often poor localization of a single focus, lack of obvious pathology and understandable surgical 'caution' in view of the proximity of the motor strip)*
- *75–85% undergoing a hemispherectomy*
- *30–40% undergoing a corpus callosotomy. (Previous practice was that the anterior two thirds would be sectioned initially, the remaining one third being cut after a further 6–12 months; current practice is that the corpus callosum should be resected completely as a 'one-step' procedure. Atonic and tonic seizures show the best response, but complex partial seizures may increase in frequency. Post-operatively, children often have a transient expressive aphasia or behavioural changes, or both)*

Outcome measures other than seizure control must also be considered, including physical functioning, concentration and learning abilities and psychosocial behaviour.[153–156] It is clear that these measures may be adversely and irreversibly affected if surgery is undertaken too late, even if seizure control is markedly improved or even complete.

Table 13
Surgical procedures for refractory seizures

Rationale	Operation	Indications
Removal of a mass of epileptogenic tissue	Standard anterior temporal lobectomy	Intractable partial epilepsy with seizure onset in the temporal lobe and normal memory function in the contralateral temporal lobe
	Selective amygdalohippocampectomy	Intractable partial epilepsy with seizure onset in medial temporal structures or when contralateral memory function is borderline
Removal of structurally abnormal tissue	Hemispherectomy*	Intractable focal ± secondary generalized seizures in patients with unilateral (static or progressive) cerebral pathology and contralateral hemiplegia with no useful hand function
	Lesionectomy	Refractory seizures due to focal pathology in resectable cortex
Disconnection procedures (separation of epileptogenic cortex from rest of brain	Corpus callosotomy	Unilateral cerebral pathology causing a focal epilepsy plus secondarily generalized seizures
	Multiple subpial transections	Intractable partial seizures originating in unresectable foci in primary cortices; may be the surgical treatment of choice for the Landau–Kleffner syndrome

*Hemispherectomy often involves both a resective and a disconnective procedure. If the entire hemisphere is anatomically removed, this may result in recognized complications, including superficial cerebral haemosiderosis and late hydrocephalus. A functional hemispherectomy is the currently preferred procedure, consisting of anatomic removal of the sensorimotor cortex and temporal lobe associated with disconnection of the remaining portions of the frontal and parieto-occipital lobes.

Vagus nerve stimulation[157–160]

The mechanism by which stimulation of the vagus nerve leads to inhibition of seizures is uncertain. Activation of pathways projecting from the nucleus solitarius of the vagus nerve to the thalami may produce an antiepileptic effect by suppressing rhythmic EEG activity. The left vagus nerve can be stimulated by a programmable generator, resembling a cardiac pacemaker, implanted beneath the left clavicle. In a multi-centre, randomized, controlled trial involving 114 subjects with intractable partial epilepsy and a mean age of 33 years, seizures were reduced by at least 50% in one third of subjects receiving active stimulation for 14 weeks, but none became seizure-free.[157] Since the first human implant in 1989, over 12 000 patients have been treated with vagus nerve stimulation (VNS), mostly in the USA and mostly in adults.[158] Efficacy amongst the growing number of subjects using VNS remains similar to the early controlled trials, with about one third showing a greater than a 50% seizure reduction, one third showing a less than 50% reduction in seizure frequency and about one third showing no significant change in seizures.

Experience of VNS in children is limited,[158,159] particularly in those with partial seizures. In an initial open study, 19 patients aged between 4 and 19 years underwent stimulation of the vagus nerve for between 2 and 30 months.[158] A 50% seizure reduction was observed in half of the subjects and a 90% reduction occurred in one third of patients (including some with the Lennox–Gastaut syndrome), with one patient becoming seizure-free. Although the number of seizures was reduced in most subjects, VNS was discontinued in over a third of subjects due to insufficient clinical improvement.

With steadily increasing experience of VNS in children, it has been found that this treatment achieves a mean seizure rate reduction of 35% in drug-resistant seizures, with results tending to be better in subjects with the Lennox–Gastaut syndrome, in whom seizure reduction rates in excess of 50% have been noted.[160]

Hoarseness during VNS is almost universal and about 10% of subjects experience coughing, although both of these complications are often temporary or respond to a reduction in the stimulation current. A tingling sensation may be felt in the neck each time that the stimulator is turned on. Importantly, there is no evidence of an increased rate of SUDEP in patients who have been implanted with a VNS device, although clearly longer-term data are required. At present, there is insufficient experience of VNS in children to justify the optimistic reports that have appeared in the general media. However, an encouraging feature emerging from adult studies is that any improvement in seizure control seems to be well maintained, and may even show further improvement, in the long term. Any benefit may not necessarily be seen until 6–12 months following VNS device implantation. It remains to be determined which seizure types (and which epilepsy syndromes) may benefit from VNS and at what age children should have the procedure.

New surgical techniques

The use of the 'gamma-knife' or 'X-knife' with precise stereotactic image guidance has improved the surgical treatment of very small lesions in eloquent (i.e. functionally important) and largely inaccessible areas of the brain. This technique is particularly effective in the management of arteriovenous malformations, cavernomas and hypothalamic hamartomas that may present with precocious puberty and drug-resistant gelastic and other, partial seizures. Gamma-knife surgery has also been used to irradiate the hippocampus in mesial temporal lobe epilepsy, with early beneficial results.

A relatively new and largely experimental technique, deep brain stimulation, is being considered for treating patients with a wide range of neurological disorders – including drug-resistant and intractable epilepsy – who are not suitable for more conventional surgical treatments. Deep brain stimulation has been used in the cerebellum, thalamic nuclei and caudate nuclei. Data are very limited and, importantly, there is no information on the longer-term outcome of patients treated with this technique. Deep brain stimulation clearly requires considerably more detailed research and evaluation.

The technique of repetitive transcranial magnetic stimulation (rTMS) in treating refractory epilepsy is also under evaluation but this is particularly experimental at the current time.

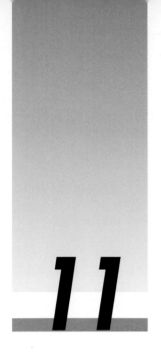

Alternative treatments of epilepsy

The indications for using alternative treatments, their efficacy and their precise modes of action have not been fully established, yet they are frequently used in children with intractable epilepsy.[161] Alternative treatments other than the ketogenic diet, steroids in infantile spasms and the epileptic encephalopathies and behaviour therapy should be considered and used with caution – and ensuring that they would not interfere with conventional antiepileptic treatments.

The ketogenic diet[161–165]

The observation that seizure frequency may be decreased during fasting often, but not invariably, at times of intercurrent illness led to the development of the ketogenic diet, which reproduces some of the metabolic effects of fasting. Ketosis is achieved by supplying the majority of dietary calories as fat, with adequate protein, carbohydrate and added vitamins and minerals to maintain nutrition. There are different types of ketogenic diet, but all are variations on a theme and as yet there is no convincing evidence that any one type is more effective and/or better tolerated than any other. Over the past decade the content and palatability of the diet have become somewhat more acceptable – to both children and their carers. The mechanism of action of the diet is unclear, but it is thought to exert an antiepileptic effect through the brain's metabolism of ketones. Myoclonic and atonic seizures respond best; the diet is used most frequently in the Lennox–Gastaut syndrome. Hospital admission is required when commencing the diet; the child is fasted for 1–2 days until ketotic. Fat, as medium-chain triglycerides (MCT), is then introduced, followed by controlled amounts of other foods. The diet requires close supervision by a dietician and also motivation from both the clinician and the child and the family. A positive response may not be seen for up to six weeks. Unfortunately, seizures may relapse even if the diet is maintained rigidly. If successful, the diet should continue for at least one or two years, during which time it may be possible to stop some, or occasionally all, of the child's antiepileptic drugs.

Although controlled trials are lacking, pooled results indicated that the ketogenic diet can achieve a greater than 50% reduction in seizures in 50–60% of children, and a greater than 90% reduction in seizures in about 30% of children. Improvement may not always be sustained in the long term, but in selected children up to 25% have shown a greater than 90% seizure reduction when the diet has been continued for at least three years. The ketogenic diet may also be a safe, and reasonably efficacious, alternative to other treatments for infantile spasms,[166] and this deserves further evaluation.

In highly selected children with epilepsy and migraine, an oligoantigenic diet may lead to an improvement in both seizure control and migraine.[167] It is not known how the diet reduces seizure frequency but this effect might relate to neurotransmitter-like substances either present in food or derived from an intestinal reaction to certain foods. Skin prick testing or IgE antibody levels are generally unhelpful in identifying foods likely to provoke seizures. Like the ketogenic diet, the oligoantigenic diet is expensive, highly demanding to maintain and requires careful medical and dietary supervision. Attempts to identify foods liable to provoke seizures in susceptible subjects (by introducing them into the diet) may rarely induce status epilepticus or anaphylaxis. Overall, the oligoantigenic diet is less useful than the ketogenic diet.

Steroids[161,168–171]

Animal studies suggest that seizures may be induced by neuronal antibodies. Although an autoimmune basis for epilepsy has not been established in humans, steroids have been prescribed for the 'intractable' childhood epilepsies, including West's syndrome, severe myoclonic epilepsy in infancy, the Lennox–Gastaut syndrome, electrical status epilepticus of slow-wave sleep (ESESS) and the Landau–Kleffner syndrome. Prednisolone (2–4 mg/kg per day) or ACTH (10–20 IU/day) is given for varying and arbitrary periods ranging from a couple of weeks to many months. In the UK, ACTH is no longer available; its 'equivalent' is tetracosactrin. ACTH is said to be superior to prednisolone because the ACTH molecule may actually function as a specific antiepileptic neuropeptide, as well as stimulating endogenous corticosteroid production[168] (the evidence for this is very limited). Steroids may suppress infantile spasms in 60–70% of infants; the effect in other epilepsies/epilepsy syndromes is less researched but would appear to be less impressive. ACTH (and tetracosactrin) have the disadvantage of requiring at least daily administration by intramuscular injection, and both ACTH and oral corticosteroids (prednisolone, betamethasone and hydrocortisone) frequently cause unpleasant and potentially serious adverse effects. It is possible that some of the side-effects seen with ACTH may be related to its preparation and formulation (including impurities, rather than the active drug). A group of neuroactive steroids with antiepileptic activity, including ganaxolone, is under development.[169] Ganaxolone is an 'epalon', a shortened form of epiallopregnanolone. Early data have suggested that it may be effective in partial seizures and infantile spasms without the side-effects seen with either ACTH or prednisolone, but further data are clearly required to assess the relative efficacy of this potentially less 'toxic' steroid.

Intravenous immunoglobulins[161,172,173]

Pooled immunoglobulins contain antibodies, directed against a variety of autoantibodies, and might theoretically be capable of 'switching off' production of putative neuronal autoantibodies. Alternatively, like steroids, immunoglobulins may have an unspecified immune effect that reduces seizure frequency. The prompt response to high-dose intravenous immunoglobulins in some patients also suggests that immunoglobulin therapy might have a direct antiepileptic action independent of any effect on the immune system. Immunoglobulin infusions have been used in the Lennox–Gastaut syndrome and other intractable epilepsies. This treatment may be most effective in some of the acute epileptic encephalopathies, including Rasmussen's encephalitis. Rasmussen's encephalitis is considered to have an autoimmune basis (involving complement-fixing anti-GluR3 antibodies) and with an onset between 18 months and 15 years of age in 80% of cases. It begins with seizures that may be insidious or, more typically, explosive. This is rapidly followed by a progressive and extremely drug-resistant partial and secondarily generalized epilepsy, with episodes of epilepsia partialis continua (that may last hours or days), and a progressive hemiplegia. High-dose immunoglobulin (doses varying from 100 to 1000 mg/kg per day) are repeated at one- to three-weekly intervals and often continued for many months. In patients without Rasmussen's encephalitis, the total duration of immunoglobulin therapy appears to be largely empirical; reports suggest that if there has been no response after three separate, consecutive doses, then it is unlikely to be effective. Children with IgG2 subclass or IgA deficiency appear to derive particular benefit, but most responders have demonstrated no obvious immune dysfunction. Immunoglobulins are expensive and carry risks (rarely) of both anaphylaxis and the transmission of blood-borne infections.

Behaviour therapy[174,175]

Behaviour therapy in the treatment of epilepsy falls into three main categories – reward/punishment approaches, self-control therapy and biofeedback techniques *(Table 14)*. More than one behavioural treatment can be used in suitable subjects. Most reports of behaviour therapy in epilepsy have been single case reports or small series and it is unclear to what extent the placebo effect contributed to any therapeutic success and whether all subjects had genuine epileptic seizures. From the few randomized trials of behaviour therapy, there is no reliable evidence of efficacy to date.[175]

Acupuncture[176-178]

Anecdotal reports of acupuncture in the treatment of epilepsy have not allowed the efficacy or indications for this treatment to be determined. A single, small controlled trial in patients with chronic intractable epilepsy did not show a significant beneficial effect of acupuncture.[176] Suppression of epileptic activity in the rat by electroacupuncture might be due to an enhancement of recurrent inhibition of the cerebral cortex and hippocampus associated with the release of various neurotransmitters, including GABA and serotonin.[176]

Herbalism, homeopathy and aromatherapy

These treatments involve, respectively, the ingestion of herbs, the ingestion of minute amounts of drugs that in larger doses would cause seizures and the use of

Table 14
Behaviour therapy in epilepsy.

Technique	Subjects	Indications
Reward/punishment	Any age and intellectual ability	1. Self-induced seizures 2. Reflex epilepsies (provoked by sensory stimuli)
Self control (including relaxation and self-abatement of seizures)	Older children and adults (difficult to apply in subjects with significant learning impairment)	1. Self-induced seizures 2. Reflex epilepsies 3. Seizures exacerbated by emotion (e.g. anxiety)
Biofeedback (self-modification of EEG)	As above	1. Reflex epilepsies 2. Seizures exacerbated by emotion

odours (aromas) to reduce seizure frequency. None of these treatments can be currently recommended in epilepsy since there have been no controlled trials to determine the efficacy of any of these treatments. Aromatherapy can be helpful in aiding relaxation as part of behaviour therapy; however, camphor, hyssop, sage and rosemary should be avoided because there is some (anecdotal) evidence that these particular substances can exacerbate seizures. Care should therefore be taken when considering these treatments because complementary medical practitioners who offer such treatments vary widely in their expertise and experience and each of these treatments has the potential to worsen epilepsy.

Status epilepticus

12

Definition, classification and aetiology[179–182]

The currently accepted definition of status epilepticus in the International Classification of Epileptic Seizures is:

'any seizure lasting for a duration of at least 30 minutes or repeated seizures lasting for 30 minutes or longer from which the patient does not regain consciousness.'

Many consider that this definition is too vague and needs revision — including specifically a reduction in the duration of a single tonic–clonic seizure from 30 to 5 minutes. The primary and most important reason for this change is to ensure that emergency or 'rescue' medication and the management of the seizure are initiated as soon as it becomes clear that the seizure has not stopped spontaneously.[183]

Any type of seizure may develop into status epilepticus; generalized tonic–clonic is the most common, and most serious, type. The current international classification of status epilepticus is likely to change under the ILAE proposals but at present the classification is as follows:

International term	Traditional term
Convulsive	
Tonic–clonic	Grand mal
Tonic or clonic	
Myoclonic	
Non-convulsive*	
Absence status	Spike and wave stupor
	'3 per second' spike and wave
	status epilepticus
	Minor status epilepticus
Partial status	
Simple	Focal motor status; epilepsia
	partialis continua
Somatomator	
Dysphasic	
Complex	Epileptic fugue state
	Prolonged epileptic stupor
	Temporal lobe status epilepticus
	Psychomotor status epilepticus
Unilateral	Hemiconvulsion–hemiplegia
	epilepsy
ESESS/CSWSS	Electrical status epilepticus of slow
	sleep [ESESS]/continuous spike
	wave of slow sleep [CSWSS]
Neonatal	

*Hypsarrhythmia is considered by many (including the authors) to be a form of non-convulsive status

The figure of 30 minutes is arbitrary and it is possible (and likely) that in the future a period of only 5 minutes may be used in any revised definition of convulsive status epilepticus. The implications for this will obviously include an earlier and more aggressive treatment of the convulsion. Consequently, the convulsion may be easier to stop (because the longer the convulsion, the more difficult it is to terminate), and importantly, there should be a reduction in status-associated mortality and morbidity.

Population-based studies suggest that the highest incidence of status epilepticus is in children and those over 60 years of age. Between 0.5% and 7% of all patients with established epilepsy will have at least one episode of status epilepticus. Although there are no precise data for the incidence and prevalence of status in children, it has been suggested that up to 70% of children with epilepsy beginning in the first year of life will experience at least one episode of status. In addition, status epilepticus is frequently the first epileptic (non-febrile) seizure in children under 3 years of age.

Diagnosis

The recognition of convulsive status is clinically obvious. The recognition of non-convulsive absence status and particularly non-convulsive complex partial status epilepticus (CPSE) may be more difficult. Absence status occurs rarely in patients with idiopathic (primary) generalized epilepsies, but complex partial status may be frequent in both symptomatic generalized (particularly Lennox-Gastaut syndrome) and symptomatic or cryptogenic partial (focal) epilepsies. Clinical manifestations of CPSE include:

- Variation in conscious level (drowsiness to stupor)
- Semi-purposeful behaviour
- Motor automatisms
- Confusion
- 'Mutism', dysphasia or dysarthria or both
- 'Ataxia' or tremulousness
- Intermittent changes in behaviour

Complex partial status in patients with learning difficulties (who may also have abnormal behaviour as part of their 'normal' profile) may be missed for days, weeks or even months. It may be misdiagnosed as a psychosis, drug intoxication or an acute encephalopathy or simply not considered. The EEG, with or without simultaneous video-monitoring, may be useful in detecting, if not diagnostic of, both absence and complex partial status. It may also be used to monitor response to treatment. Where there is a clinical suspicion of non-convulsive status, an EEG must be undertaken.

Non-convulsive status may also be over-diagnosed (or at least overly considered), again particularly in children with learning difficulties or behavioural problems, or both. In these situations the differential diagnosis includes:

- Antiepileptic drug toxicity (acute or chronic); other drug intoxication
- Prolonged post-ictal state (i.e. a confusional state)
- An organic encephalopathy (e.g. metabolic disorder, including hypoglycaemia or lead poisoning; hydrocephalus; cerebral tumour)
- A dementing disorder (including degenerative conditions such as SSPE or Huntington's disease or variant Creutzfeldt–Jakob disease)
- Psychiatric disorder (including a bipolar depression or disintegrative psychosis)

Rarely, non-convulsive status may be converted into convulsive (particularly tonic) status by benzodiazepines.

Aetiology[180,184–187]

The causes of status epilepticus are multiple and can be divided generally into:

> - Remote symptomatic (where there is a chronic non-progressive or progressive disturbance of brain function, including epilepsy)
>
> - Acute symptomatic (acute neurological or systemic disorder, including infections – meningitis and encephalitis – and metabolic disorders)
>
> - Febrile (occurring in febrile children with no previous history of non-febrile seizures and no evidence of meningitis/encephalitis)
>
> - Idiopathic (cryptogenic)

The majority of paediatric status is symptomatic (acute or remote), and there is a close correlation with age. A comparison of causes in children and adults appears in *Table 15*.

Febrile seizures are the major cause of acute 'idiopathic' status. Whether these are truly 'idiopathic' remains to be determined with earlier and more sensitive imaging techniques (see Chapter 6 on Febrile seizures). Up to 5–10% of children with a first febrile seizure will present with febrile status epilepticus. Acute anticonvulsant withdrawal as a cause of status is more common in the teenager or adolescent than in the younger child – and is certainly one of the most common cause of convulsive status epilepticus in teenagers and young adults. Pseudo-epileptic status (i.e. non-epileptic status epilepticus) occurs rarely in the paediatric population, but not infrequently begins to emerge as a phenomenon in teenage girls between 13 and 16 years of age and is relatively common in young adults, and often in those who also have mild learning difficulties.

Table 15
Causes of status epilepticus.

Causes	Children <16 years (%)	Adults > 16 years (%)
Fever/infection	35.7	4.6
Medication change	19.8	18.9
Unknown ('idiopathic')	9.3	8.1
Metabolic	8.2	8.8
Congenital	7.0	0.8
Anoxia	5.3	10.7
CNS infection	4.8	1.8
Trauma	3.5	4.6
Cerebrovascular	3.3	25.2
Ethanol/drug-related	2.4	12.2
Tumour	0.7	4.3

(Modified from Pellock[179] based on a study of De Lorenzo et al[182] in 171 children and 375 adults.)

Pathophysiology

Numerous studies in both animals and man have demonstrated that prolonged convulsive status (longer than 60, and possibly longer than 30 minutes) may cause irreversible neuronal damage within the hippocampus, amygdala, cerebellum and thalamus, and even the cerebral cortex. This damage may occur in the absence of any metabolic dysfunction, including hypoxia and hypoglycaemia, and results from a cytotoxic chain reaction involving excitatory amino acids (e.g. glutamate), free-radical release, mitochondrial dysfunction, cerebral oedema and cerebral ischaemia. Persisting status epilepticus leads to a loss of physiological compensatory mechanisms, with consequent biochemical, renal, hepatic and cardiac failure, and, ultimately, death.

Mortality and long-term sequelae[185–187]

The mortality of children with status epilepticus has improved considerably over the past 15 years, from approximately 10% in 1970, to under 4% in 1989. Morbidity (including irreversible neurological damage) has improved from over 50% (1970) to 10% (1989). These better outcomes reflect a combination of a more rapid diagnosis and treatment of

status and improved intensive care facilities. The more refractory and drug-resistant the episodes of status, the greater the mortality rate, and this is related predominantly to the cause and age of the child rather than the duration of the status – although the duration of status may contribute to any secondary cerebral 'damage'.

In children both mortality and morbidity are also related to the underlying cause, being more common in symptomatic rather than febrile or 'idiopathic' cases. Importantly, febrile status epilepticus does not appear to increase the risk of further febrile or afebrile (i.e. epileptic) seizures. Finally, prolonged non-convulsive status (usually complex partial) may also cause long-term sequelae, including memory and other cognitive impairment.

Treatment[180–182,185–187]

Convulsive and non-convulsive status epilepticus are medical and neurological emergencies. In convulsive status the time-interval between onset of seizures and the start of effective therapy (as well as the underlying cause) is important in determining the prognosis, largely through preventing any secondary brain damage.

Management includes:

- Maintaining a patent airway and adequate cardiorespiratory function

- Correct positioning of the child

- Identifying and treating any precipitating factors

- Stopping the seizure as quickly as possible

- Preventing any secondary brain damage by maintaining homeostasis (tissue oxygenation, fluid and electrolyte balance, normoglycaemia, blood pressure, etc.) – these issues are frequently neglected but are very important, particularly in prolonged status, and may contribute to or even cause additional irreversible cerebral damage if ignored

- Preventing seizure recurrence

Current accepted practice is to use an intravenous short-acting benzodiazepine (lorazepam or diazepam) bolus first and then to give a second dose if the seizure continues *(Figure 22)*. In the UK, intravenous lorazepam is the currently preferred benzodiazepine in the management of an acute tonic–clonic convulsion and status epilepticus.[188–190] If status persists or a seizure recurs within 10–15 minutes then the child should be given rectal paraldehyde and intravenous phenytoin. Although paraldehyde may be given as an intramuscular injection (1 ml per year of age up to a maximum of 6 ml), this may damage the sciatic nerve and cause sterile abscesses; the preferred route is rectal (0.4 ml/kg with 0.4 ml/kg paraffin or mineral oil). Paraldehyde is well absorbed from the rectum and is frequently effective when diazepam has failed.

In infants and young children venous access may be difficult, and to avoid unnecessary delay, rectal administration of a benzodiazepine (diazepam, 0.5 mg/kg or lorazepam 0.1 mg/kg)[191] or paraldehyde should be given rapidly. Absorption is good and effective blood levels are achieved relatively quickly.

Phenytoin is arguably preferable to phenobarbitone as the first long-acting anticonvulsant; the latter may cause respiratory depression (or arrest), particularly if given after a benzodiazepine or paraldehyde, and hypotension which may exacerbate cerebral ischaemia and therefore the mortality/morbidity of status. The risk of causing a cardiac arrhythmia with phenytoin is low and can be avoided by ensuring that the rate of infusion is no greater than 1 mg/kg per minute. The initial 'loading' dose of phenytoin is 18 mg/kg and phenobarbitone 20 mg/kg; a serum level should be measured approximately 1 hour after the infusion is completed to ensure a 'therapeutic' level has been achieved and to determine the timing and amount of subsequent maintenance doses.

If status persists, the child must be stabilized first and then transferred to intensive care, principally to provide cardiorespiratory support and to prevent/minimize any secondary medical complications.

Status persisting on admission to intensive care requires barbiturate

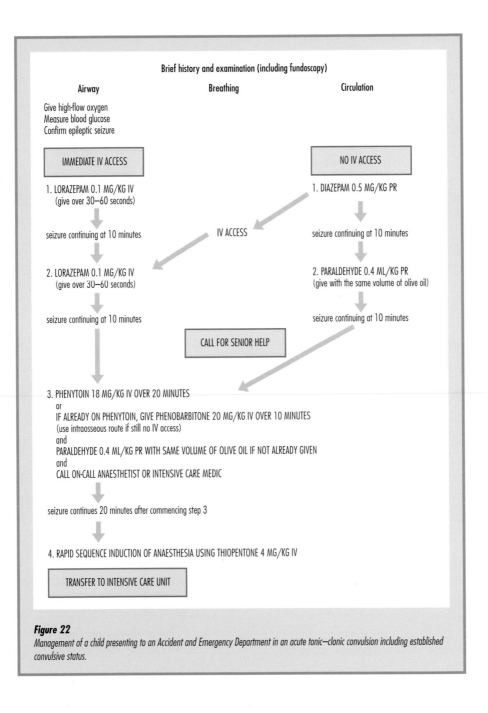

Figure 22
Management of a child presenting to an Accident and Emergency Department in an acute tonic–clonic convulsion including established convulsive status.

anaesthesia (usually with thiopentone) and cerebral protective measures. EEG monitoring (with standard EEG or with continuous cerebral function analysis monitoring – CFAM) is useful in monitoring convulsive and non-convulsive status, particularly when the child has received neuromuscular blockade (paralysis), or whenever seizure recurrence cannot be documented clinically.

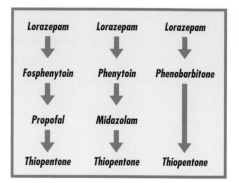

Other drugs that may be of benefit in convulsive status include:

- Paraldehyde (a continuous infusion may also be used: 1–3 ml/kg per hour of a 5% solution ensuring that all tubing used in the infusion set is 'protected' from sunlight)

- Lignocaine (5 mg/kg bolus; 4–6 mg/kg per hour infusion)

- Diazepam (0.1–0.4 mg/kg per hour infusion)

- Midazolam (0.15 mg/kg bolus; 0.06–0.6 mg/kg per hour infusion)

- Clonazepam (0.25–0.5 mg or 0.05 mg/kg bolus; infusion rarely used)

Intravenous sodium valproate has also been reported (rarely) to be of benefit in treating convulsive status and acute, frequent repeated seizures.[192]

In many units and particularly in the USA, different treatment regimes and 'cascades' are used other than that outlined in *Figure 22*. Some of these regimes include:

(It must be emphasized that the vast majority of protocols for treating convulsive status in children are based predominantly on anecdotal and clinical experience, rather than being 'evidence-based', i.e. based on randomized clinical and comparative trials.)

Additional routes are being evaluated for giving short- but rapidly acting anticonvulsants.[193–196] In part this reflects the concern that has been expressed by a number of teachers, hospice staff and even some childrens' carers/parents with using the rectal route in giving the currently most commonly prescribed 'rescue' or emergency medication – diazepam. Intranasal (or buccal) midazolam (in a dose of 0.2 mg/kg) is 'well' absorbed and it has been reported to be of benefit,[194–196] primarily for treating repeated serial seizures; its effect in established convulsive status epilepticus has yet to be formally assessed. The results of a national multicentre randomized clinical trial comparing rectal diazepam with buccal midazolam in approximately 200 children presenting to

Accident and Emergency Departments in an acute tonic–clonic convulsion may determine whether buccal midazolam should replace rectal diazepam as the first-choice 'rescue' or emergency drug in treating acute tonic–clonic seizures (results are expected from the authors in 2004). The buccal route may have clear practical and 'ethical' advantages over the rectal route – and this would reasonably support the use of midazolam in preference to diazepam as the preferred rescue drug for non-hospital use – including for use at home, in special schools and by paramedic ambulance staff. The authors' current preferred non-rectal route for midazolam is buccal rather than intranasal.

In the USA, fosphenytoin has replaced phenytoin as the first-choice, long-acting drug used in convulsive status epilepticus.[197–199] Fosphenytoin is water-soluble and is therefore less irritant to veins and tissues. The drug may also be infused more rapidly than phenytoin, apparently with less risk of causing cardiac arrhythmias, although the Committee on Safety of Medicines in the UK has received reports of cardiac arrhythmias and hypotension. Fosphenytoin is also prescribed as phenytoin equivalents (which can result in prescribing errors) and the drug is currently five times more expensive than phenytoin. The risk of tissue necrosis and cardiac arrhythmias with intravenous phenytoin may be more potential than real, providing the drug is administered with care, using recommended guidelines.[200]

The treatments of non-convulsive and convulsive status are similar; non-convulsive status tends to be more resistant to treatment (particularly to benzodiazepines), and frequently recurs even after initial control.

As stated previously, benzodiazepines may occasionally convert non-convulsive status into convulsive (tonic or tonic–clonic) status, particularly in children with difficult epilepsies, including the Lennox–Gastaut syndrome. In refractory or recurrent complex partial or absence status additional drugs or procedures may sometimes be effective:

- Prednisolone/hydrocortisone (particularly for absence or myoclonic status; although the response to steroids may be transient, it may also be sustained and 'switch off' the status for some considerable time, particularly if the maintenance dose of the steroid is given for at least 2–4 weeks and then withdrawn very gradually)

- Lamotrigine (although the main disadvantage with this drug is its required slow gradual introduction over a few weeks because of the risk of rash)

- Topiramate (a positive response may be seen within 5–7 days)

- Intravenous immunoglobulins

- Ketogenic diet (although it is likely to take a minimum of 21 days before any positive response may be seen)

- 'Urgent' functional hemispherectomy (e.g. Rasmussen's encephalitis)

The impact of epilepsy

13

Social implications of epilepsy

Relatively few restrictions are necessary for children with epilepsy, and they should be encouraged to participate in and enjoy a full social life.[201] Perhaps not unsurprisingly, it has been found that the importance of restrictions may in part be determined by doctors' own attitudes and beliefs in this area.[202] Parents frequently ask the doctor to arbitrate or decide what activity their child should and should not be allowed to do – and this particularly relates to the use of play stations and playing of video-games on personal computers. Epileptic seizures are less likely to occur when an individual is engaged in satisfying mental or physical activity. Clearly, certain activities do require a specific comment:

- Domestic bathing (young children should always be supervised and older children should shower or use a shallow bath, keeping the bathroom door unlocked)

- Swimming (a competent adult swimmer should be available on the pool-side or close to the water-side for any child with epilepsy)[203]

- Horse-riding and cycling (a helmet should always be used for both activities [irrespective of whether the child has epilepsy] and busy roads should be avoided)

- In most situations, the unsupervised climbing of trees and rocks should be avoided unless the seizures are well controlled

- There is no obvious medical reason why children with epilepsy should not be allowed to participate in most if not all of the rides and activities at adventure playgrounds and theme parks

- Most children and teenagers with epilepsy are not photosensitive and should experience no difficulties with any computer work, including video-games, and should not be excluded from information technology courses at schools and colleges

There is a complicated relationship between sleep and epilepsy.[204] Some seizures and epilepsy syndromes are more common during, or exclusive to, sleep. Disorders of sleep, particularly sleep apnoea, can co-exist with epilepsy and seizures may independently interfere with normal sleep. Excessive drowsiness is often attributed to either medication or poorly controlled epilepsy, but more detailed sleep studies should be considered since various sleep disorders (specifically narcolepsy and obstructive sleep apnoea) requiring specific management may be the primary cause of drowsiness. Although sleep deprivation has long been believed to exacerbate seizures, there is surprisingly little evidence to support this assumption; however, doctors and most young people with epilepsy would accept that it is a real effect!

Teenagers attending discotheques or concerts are at a low risk of low-frequency stroboscopic lighting-induced seizures. Driving restrictions for those with epilepsy have been gradually liberalized, but currently vary widely around the world and even from state to state within the USA.[205] In the UK, teenagers aged 17 years and above may learn to drive if *either* they have had no epileptic seizures for the past year *or* they have only had epileptic seizures while asleep for the previous three years. This information forewarns those with poor seizure control that they will not be permitted to drive, enables those with complete seizure control to decide if and when to withdraw medication and, finally, may motivate some adolescents to comply with their medication. It is important to tell the teenager that these driving regulations apply irrespective of whether or not they are taking antiepileptic medication. If a teenager is already driving and wants to discontinue any antiepileptic medication, they should be advised to stop driving whilst the drug is withdrawn (slowly over at least six or eight weeks) and for a further six months after the drug has been discontinued. Driving can then be resumed if there has been no seizure recurrence.

Adolescents also require counselling and advice about employment; this is important because any early enthusiasm for certain prohibited occupations, e.g. the armed services, piloting commercial aircraft, the ambulance, police and fire services and driving public transport vehicles, can be channelled towards other careers. Despite an increased scientific interest, there is still a considerable misunderstanding of epilepsy, and, therefore, an unfair prejudice towards, and a stigmatization of, people (including children) with this condition. There are no automatic restrictions or barriers to most other professions or employment, and these include:

- medicine, nursing and allied health professions (occupational, speech and physiotherapy)
- law
- accountancy
- teaching (schools, colleges, universities)

- hairdressing
- shop assistant; shop keeping
- clerical, secretarial and administrative
- business and information technology

Further specific advice on career and employment opportunities can be obtained from the relevant career information advisers (including 'Connexions') and disability resettlement officers. The Disability Discrimination Act of 1995, with more extensive reinforcement within the past 12–18 months, has been very helpful in establishing rights and support for young people with epilepsy and assisting them in securing appropriate employment.

The unemployment rate amongst young adults who had epilepsy during childhood is reassuringly low, although the rate is higher than found in the general population. Social immaturity and a more dependent life-style tends to be more common in young adults who had experienced epilepsy in childhood. However, these social difficulties are much more common in those who also have learning difficulties, and are not independently related either to having had epilepsy in childhood or to the need to continue taking antiepileptic drugs through into adulthood.[206]

Psychological implications of epilepsy[207–211]

The unpredictability (not knowing when a seizure may occur), together with the sudden loss of control that typifies most seizures, is distressing for patients and their friends and carers. A simple explanation of epilepsy lessens the psychological impact on those who are likely to witness seizures. Understandably, parents tend to over-protect children with epilepsy, but this should be sympathetically discouraged, but in doing so, the family must be offered help, advice and support as to how they can do this. The psychological effect of epilepsy on a child depends on a number of factors, including:

- The child's personality
- Seizure type and epilepsy syndrome
- Effectiveness and side-effects of treatment
- Any additional health problems
- Relationship with health care professionals
- Attitude of their school, family and friends

Unfortunately, behavioural difficulties in children with epilepsy are not uncommon, particularly in the teenage years, in view of the additional emotional difficulties that are prevalent at this time of life. A significant number may suffer a loss of self-esteem, anxiety or depression, requiring formal psychological or psychiatric support. There is some evidence that behavioural problems may pre-exist before the onset of seizures[212] although this may be dependent on the type and cause of the epilepsy.

Psychiatric disorders occur more frequently with epilepsy than with other chronic disorders; the highest rate of disturbance is found in children with symptomatic and temporal lobe epilepsy.

Cognitive impairment in children with complex partial seizures is related to early age at onset of recurrent seizures, whereas behavioural disturbances appear to be more closely related to recent seizure frequency.[210]

The psychological impact of epilepsy is being increasingly studied using quality-of-life and behavioural measures as part of outcome assessments in trials of antiepileptic drugs. However, a variety of outcome measures are used in such studies and care must be taken to choose measurement tools that are relevant and appropriate to populations with epilepsy.[213]

Finally, it is important to emphasize that there is no such phenomenon as the 'epileptic personality'; any child or teenager with a chronic disease, and particularly one that is unpredictable and potentially frightening as epilepsy, is at risk of developing some stereotypical behaviour patterns.

Educational implications of epilepsy[202,210,214–217]

The potential social and psychological effects of epilepsy may also have significant educational consequences. Families should be encouraged to discuss their child's seizures with school staff so that teachers are prepared for the possible occurrence of seizures in the classroom or on the school playing field and in the swimming pool. Children are highly adaptable, and will understand a classmate's seizure if an accurate explanation of the seizure and the child's behaviour is given, and provided that the class teacher does not appear frightened or upset. Conversely children may be very cruel and may subject their classmate with epilepsy to teasing and bullying. This is particularly a problem in secondary rather than primary school; it is therefore important to educate and inform children about the facts of epilepsy sooner rather than later – and certainly within primary schools. Teachers' knowledge of epilepsy is generally good, although they are apprehensive about the practical management of this condition, indicating a need for improved liaison between health and education services. A teacher should be able to provide basic first aid for a pupil having a seizure. A school nurse may administer rectal diazepam to a child experiencing a prolonged convulsion, although this is only likely to be required in relatively few children, and particularly in special schools.

With the exception of epilepsy syndromes associated with progressive neurological disease, the majority of children with epilepsy do not experience progressive deterioration of intellect. The measured IQ of a child with epilepsy may sometimes appear to fall with increasing age. This is occasionally referred to as 'pseudo-dementia'; in the vast majority of cases this is due to intellectual skills advancing more slowly than normal with increasing age, rather than representing a true reduction in, or loss of, intellect.

Learning difficulties, either general or specific, are not uncommon in children with epilepsy. There may be many reasons why children with epilepsy may experience learning difficulties:

- Any underlying structural lesion (e.g. tuberous sclerosis, polymicrogyria, following an acquired brain injury)

- Unrecognized and frequent seizures (including episodes of non-convulsive status epilepticus)

- Frequent subclinical epileptiform activity (usually occurring over many months/years); this may include the Landau–Kleffner syndrome and electrical status epilepticus of slow-wave sleep (ESESS)

- Toxic effects of antiepileptic medication

- Emotional and psychological influences (at home, amongst peers and at school – these are frequently ignored or under-recognized – but should always be considered)

- Familial/genetic trait (e.g. fragile X syndrome)

- Rarely, an underlying progressive degenerative (and dementing) disorder

---

More commonly, it is a combination of these factors, rather than a single factor, that gives rise to significant learning difficulties in children with epilepsy. Importantly, similar factors are responsible for many of the behavioural problems that may also occur in children who do not have epilepsy but some other chronic medical condition.

Seizure activity itself, particularly frequent temporal lobe or absence seizures, subclinical epileptiform activity or non-convulsive status, may contribute to learning difficulties. Adverse effects from certain antiepileptic drugs must also be considered. Close liaison is required between health and educational professionals in the identification and assessment of learning difficulties in children with epilepsy. Fortunately, most (60–70%) are able to be educated in mainstream school (although some experience frequent seizures); a minority require special schooling because of additional physical/learning problems, and less than 1% attend special (often residential) schools for epilepsy. With the increasing focus on social integration or social inclusion for children with special educational needs (including children with epilepsy) into mainstream schools, this should (at least theoretically) increase everyone's (teachers', pupils' and parents') knowledge and understanding of epilepsy. It should also facilitate and enable the child with epilepsy to participate in and contribute to all the activities within their school. This is the theory; the authors hope that this becomes a reality and that it is put into practice.

Administering rectal diazepam may be considered socially unacceptable in school, or elsewhere outside a hospital, to the point where some schools have refused to administer the drug and have insisted that either the parents come in to give the drug or the child be admitted to hospital – both of which are inappropriate and unnecessary. Buccal or intranasal midazolam has been found to be at least as effective as rectal diazepam for the treatment of prolonged seizures in a special school setting,[194–196,218] and studies are in progress to determine whether buccal midazolam is acceptable and effective in less specialized schools and in other settings outside hospital.

Epilepsy clinics

The management of epilepsy extends far beyond the identification of the specific epilepsy syndrome/seizure type and the underlying cause and the prescription of the most appropriate antiepileptic drug. For many patients (particularly children) and their families, social, educational and psychological problems are more important than simply controlling the seizures. Ideally, this requires a multidisciplinary or 'team' approach, preferably within a specialist clinic, with education, support and advice from many different sources.[219] Members of this team should include the following, of whom an experienced doctor and nurse specialist are probably the key people:

- Dedicated medical staff (interested and experienced in childhood epilepsy)
- Nurse specialist in paediatric epilepsy
- Clinical psychologist
- Social worker
- Representative(s) of the local or national voluntary epilepsy associations

---

Opponents of an epilepsy or seizure clinic (who, fortunately are in a minority) consider that they serve only to further stigmatize and isolate these children, when in fact the reverse is true. Clinics for other chronic childhood disorders, including diabetes, asthma and cystic fibrosis, are well established and are considered the best format and environment for managing these children. Although epilepsy is far more heterogeneous than these other conditions this does not, and should not, preclude it from having its own specific clinic.

The purposes of the clinic are multiple, providing not only the best medical assessment/treatment, but also a service that offers information, education, counselling and psychological support. This could include identifying the most effective and appropriate way of telling children and their families about epilepsy and describing what exactly 'seizures', 'fits' and epilepsy mean.[220] The clinic environment and staff provide a focused and concentrated resource of expertise. The clinic should also maximize the potential for listening to the family (and their child) about their needs and concerns. It cannot be over-emphasized that the families of children with epilepsy are themselves 'experts' – in having to live with, and cope with epilepsy, particularly when their child has additional physical, learning or behavioural problems. The specialist clinic staff should be able to listen and to understand – and then try and address these needs and concerns.

Where possible there should be a separate clinic for teenagers with epilepsy, for whom follow-up in a children's hospital or unit is no longer appropriate (see Chapter 7 on Epilepsy in adolescence). The epilepsy clinic may be sited in any paediatric unit or children's hospital; it should not be exclusive to a teaching or referral centre. However, it is important that the clinic should not exist in isolation within the hospital; one of the key purposes of the clinic is to form a close link or liaison between the hospital and community health services (including school health and general practice), the hospital and the family, and the hospital and the school (specifically teachers), and in doing so to attempt to reduce the unfortunate 'sick' or 'illness' stigma which is so often (inappropriately) associated with epilepsy.

The clinical nurse specialist[221–223] in epilepsy would clearly be the pivotal team member in establishing the all-important hospital–community and hospital–family links (through school and home visits) and providing a management and education framework for the primary health care teams. A nurse is often regarded as being a less threatening and generally more approachable person than a doctor, and is therefore more readily able to understand and be understood by families and children, particularly teenagers. A nurse may be able to obtain valuable information following home visits that may have a direct influence on the management of the child (e.g. in identifying that compliance with medication is poor, that the teenager may be taking recreational drugs, that a girl may be sexually active or even pregnant – or that there is major marital/parental discord). Although it is difficult to prove the benefit or cost-effectiveness of the nurse specialist,[222,223] there is a broad consensus that the provision of this resource and their input is generally important in improving the holistic management of people (of all ages) with epilepsy. This has been highlighted in a number of reports[224,225] and consensus statements, including the Clinical Standards Advisory Group (CSAG), commissioned by the Department of Health to evaluate services for children and adults with epilepsy throughout the UK.[225]

For far too long epilepsy has been 'in the shadows', the name given to the global campaign in 1997 launched by the World Health Organization to address the inadequacy of care in epilepsy. This relates to not only the inadequacy of epilepsy care, but also the limited availability of both appropriate and enthusiastic medical training and clinically relevant research as well as inadequate Government awareness and unacceptable public stigmatization. There is some evidence that the shadows are shortening and light is dawning; one can only hope that this is not yet another 'false dawn'.

Appendix 1

Key points on childhood epilepsy

- Epilepsy is a clinical diagnosis based on a detailed history; if there is any doubt, do not diagnose epilepsy – and wait and see; re-take the history and obtain video-recordings of the child's episodes
- Make every attempt to obtain the history or account of the child's or adolescent's episodes from an eye witness and not just 'second-hand'
- Always ask the child or teenager themselves about **their** memory of the episodes (before, during and after the episode)
- Use the EEG to classify the epilepsy syndrome and not to diagnose epilepsy
- Epilepsy affects 0.6–0.7% of all school-age children
- Up to 70–75% of childhood epilepsy will have no identified cause
- Children with infantile spasms, with simple and complex partial seizures, and with epilepsy and developmental regression require brain imaging
- Sodium valproate (generalized seizures) and carbamazepine (partial seizures) are currently the drugs of first choice for the majority of the childhood epilepsies; topiramate and lamotrigine may be useful alternatives for either partial or generalized tonic–clonic seizures
- Carbamazepine exacerbates myoclonic and typical absence seizures, including causing myoclonic or

absence status, and exacerbates spike/polyspike and slow-wave activity on the EEG

- Families should be provided with written information on the type and prognosis of the epilepsy syndrome, side-effects of the anticonvulsants and the name and address of a voluntary epilepsy association
- There is no indication for the routine measurement of serum levels of antiepileptic drugs; levels should be measured where there is suspicion of major non-compliance with medication or if the child presents in status epilepticus
- Children who are considered to have a benign partial or generalized epilepsy syndrome but whose seizures remain poorly controlled should be considered to be possibly non-compliant with their antiepileptic medication
- Children in whom the diagnosis of their paroxysmal episodes is unclear or uncertain should be discussed with or referred to a paediatric neurologist
- Children with poor seizure control require referral to a specialist in paediatric epilepsy (i.e. a paediatric neurologist); epilepsy surgery should be considered early and within 2 years of presentation if seizures are frequent and/or drug-resistant
- Children and teenagers with epilepsy should be managed in an epilepsy clinic with access to a nurse specialist in epilepsy
- If the child has been seizure-free for 18 months to 2 years on antiepileptic medication, consideration should be given to withdrawing the drug in full discussion with the family and, when appropriate, the child or teenager
- In most situations an antiepileptic drug can be withdrawn over 6–8 weeks; unless the child is likely to remain in hospital for some weeks, withdrawal should rarely take place over less than 4 weeks
- Children/teenagers with epilepsy, irrespective of seizure control and whether they are receiving an antiepileptic drug, should remain under paediatric/paediatric neurology review until **either** the antiepileptic drug has been successfully withdrawn and they have remained seizure-free for at least 6–12 months after the drug has been discontinued, **or** their care has been transferred to an adult neurologist with an interest in epilepsy
- Communication at all levels and between all professionals involved with the child and their family is fundamental for optimal epilepsy care; this clearly must include listening to the child and family about any concerns and issues.

Appendix 2

Medico-legal aspects of epilepsy

Not unexpectedly, there are a number of diagnostic and management issues that may have potential and significant medico-legal implications. Many of these issues have already resulted in successful litigation for the plaintiff. These issues include:

- establishing the correct diagnosis of epilepsy or another paroxysmal but non-epileptic disorder
- recognizing and treating electrical or non-convulsive status epilepticus
- recognizing and diagnosing infantile spasms and hypsarrhythmia on the EEG
- ensuring that an underlying cause for the epilepsy has always been considered – and appropriately investigated (e.g. relevant biochemical [specifically glucose, sodium and calcium in infants and young children] and neuroimaging investigations)
- ensuring that the most appropriate antiepileptic drug has been prescribed for the correct seizure type and epilepsy syndrome (e.g. **not** prescribing carbamazepine or phenytoin for childhood or juvenile-onset absence and juvenile myoclonic epilepsies)
- appropriately managing convulsive status epilepticus as a medical emergency
- giving appropriate advice to families about the

relevant and potentially serious side-
effects or drug interactions with some
of the antiepileptic drugs (e.g. rashes
with carbamazepine and lamotrigine;
liver dysfunction in neonates and
infants with sodium valproate; visual
field constriction with vigabatrin; renal
stones with topiramate; the reduced
effect of the oral contraceptive pill
with carbamazepine and topiramate;
the increased risk of Reye's syndrome
or bleeding with sodium valproate and
aspirin)

- giving appropriate advice regarding the
potential effects of antiepileptic drugs
on the fetus before any pregnancy, and
certainly if the young person is
sexually active
- giving accurate and appropriate advice
about possible restrictions in career
choice
- giving accurate advice about the
current driving regulations
- giving appropriate advice about the
increased risks of death that may
rarely occur in certain types of
epilepsy and certain causes of
epilepsy

Appendix 3

Useful addresses and contact details (as of September 2003)

'Brainwave'
The Irish Epilepsy Association
249 Crumlin Road
Dublin 12
Ireland

Tel: 00 353 1 455 7500
Fax: 00 353 1 455 7013
Website: www.epilepsy.ie
E-mail: info@epilepsy.ie

Employment Medical Advisory Service
Health and Safety Executive
EMAS (London Division)
Rosecourt
2 Southwark Bridge
London SE1 9HS

Tel: 020 7556 2100
Fax: 020 7556 2109
Website: www.hse.gov.uk

Epilepsy Action (formerly British Epilepsy Association)
New Anstey house
Gateway Drive
Yeadon
Leeds LS19 7XY

Tel: 0113 210 8800
Fax: 0113 391 0300
Helpline: Freephone 0808 800 5050
Website: www.epilepsy.org.uk
E-mail: epilepsy@epilepsy.org.uk

Epilepsy Bereaved
PO Box 112
Wantage
Oxon, OX12 8XT

Tel/Fax: 01235 772 850
Bereavement Contact Line: 01235 772852
Website: www.sudep.org
E-mail: epilepsybereaved@dial.pipex.com

Epilepsy Action Scotland
48 Govan Road
Glasgow G51 1JL

Tel: 0141 427 4911
Fax: 0141 419 1709
Website: www.epilepsyscotland.org.uk
E-mail: enquiries@epilepsyscotland.org.uk
Helpline: 0808 800 2200

Epilepsy Canada
Suite 745
1470 Peel Street
Montreal
Quebec
Canada H3A 1T1

Tel: 001 514 845 7855
Website: www.epilepsy.ca

Epilepsy Foundation of America
4351 Garden City Drive
Landover
Maryland 20785-7223
USA

Tel: 001 800 332 1000
Website: www.epilepsyfoundation.org

Epilepsy Research Foundation
PO Box 3004
London W4 1XT

Tel/Fax: 0208 995 4781
Website: www.erf.org.uk
E-mail: info@erf.org.uk

Epilepsy Wales
15 Chester Street
St Asaph
Denbighshire LL17 0RE

Helpline: 0845 741 3774
Tel/Fax: 01745 584444
Website: www.epilepsy-wales.co.uk
E-mail: office@epilepsy-wales.co.uk

International Bureau for Epilepsy
IBE
Achterweg 5
2103 SW Heemstede
The Netherlands

Tel: 0031 235 291019

MedicAlert
No.1 Bridge Wharf
156 Caledonian Road
London N1 9UU

Tel: 020 7833 3034
Fax: 020 7278 0647
Website: www.medicalert.org.uk
E-mail: membership@medicalert.org.uk

Mersey Region Epilepsy Association
Glaxo Neurological Centre
Norton Street
Liverpool L3 8LR

Tel: 0151 298 2666
Fax: 0151 298 2333
Website: www.epilepsymersey.org.uk
E-mail: epilepsy@mrea.demon.co.uk

National Society for Epilepsy
Chesham Lane
Chalfont St Peter
Buckinghamshire SL9 0RJ

Tel: 01494 601300
Fax: 01494 871927
Helpline: 01494 601400
Website: www.epilepsynse.org.uk

References

1 Jackson JH (1873). On the anatomical, physiological and pathological investigation of epilepsies. West Riding Lunatic Asylum Medical Reports 3. 3.5. Reprinted in: Taylor J (ed). *Selected Writing of John Hughlings Jackson*. Sevenoaks, Kent: Hodder and Stoughton, 1983: 90–111.

2 Anderson VE, Hauser WA and Rich SS. Genetic heterogeneity in the epilepsies. In: Delgado-Escueta AV, Ward Jr AA, Woodbury DM and Porter RJ (eds). *Advances in Neurology 44*. New York: Raven Press, 1986.

3 Hauser WA and Kurland LT. The epidemiology of epilepsy in Rochester, Minnesota, 1935 through 1967. *Epilepsia* 1975; **16:** 1–66.

4 Harvey AS, Nolan T and Carlin JB. Community-based study of mortality in children with epilepsy. *Epilepsia* 1993; **34:** 597–603.

5 Callenbach PMC, Westendorp RGJ, Geerts AT et al. Mortality risk in children with epilepsy: the Dutch study of epilepsy in childhood. *Pediatrics* 2001; **107:** 1259–63.

6 Camfield CS, Camfield PR and Vengelers PJ. Death in children with epilepsy: a population-based study. *Lancet* 2002; **359:** 1891–5.

7 Hauser WA, Annegers JF and Elveback LR. Mortality in patients with epilepsy. *Epilepsia* 1980; **21:** 399–412.

8 Kurokawa T, Funs KC, Hanai T and Goya N. Mortality and clinical features in cases of death among epileptic children. *Brain Dev* 1982; **4–5:** 321–5.

9 Jay GW and Leetsma JE. Sudden death in epilepsy. *Acta Neurol Scand* 1981; **63 (Suppl 82):** 1–66.

10 Leetsma JE, Walczak T, Hughes JR, Kalelkar MB and Teas SS. A prospective study on sudden unexpected death in epilepsy. *Ann Neurol* 1989; **26:** 195–203.

11 Hanna NJ, Black M, Sander JWS et al. *The National Sentinel Clinical Audit of Epilepsy-Related Death.* London: The Stationery Office, 2002.

12 Appleton RE. Mortality in paediatric epilepsy. *Arch Dis Child* 2004; (In press).

13 Gibbs J and Appleton RE. False diagnosis of epilepsy in children. *Seizure* 1992; **1**: 15–18.

14 Aicardi J. Paroxysmal disorders other than epilepsy. In: *Diseases of the Nervous System in Childhood, Clinics in Developmental Medicine Nos 115–118.* London: MacKeith Press, 1992: 1001–38.

15 Daley HM and Appleton RE. Fits, faints and funny turns. *Current Paediatrics* 2000; **10**: 22–7.

16 Jeavons PM. The practical management of epilepsy. *Update* 1975; **1**: 11–15.

17 Kinsbourne M. Hiatus hernia with contortions of the neck. *Lancet* 1964; **i**: 1058–61.

18 Holmes GL and Russman BS. Shuddering attacks. *Am J Dis Child* 1986; **140**: 72–4.

19 Meadow R. Munchhausen syndrome by proxy. *Arch Dis Child* 1982; **57**: 92–8.

20 Meadow R. Fictitious epilepsy. *Lancet* 1984; **ii**: 25–8.

21 Carmant L, Kramer U, Holmes GL et al. Differential diagnosis of staring spells in children: A video-EEG study. *Pediatr Neurol* 1996; **14**: 199–202.

22 McLeod KA. Syncope in childhood. *Arch Dis Child* 2003: **88**: 350–3.

23 Stephenson JBP. Reflex anoxic seizures ('white breath-holding') non-epileptic vagal attacks. *Arch Dis Child* 1978; **53**: 193–200.

24 Lancman ME, Asconape JJ, Graves S and Gibson PA. Psychogenic seizures in children: long-term analysis of 43 cases. *J Child Neurol* 1994; **9**: 404–7.

25 Irwin K, Edwards M and Robinson R. Psychogenic non-epileptic seizures: management and prognosis. *Arch Dis Child* 2000; **82**: 474–8.

26 Gudmundsson O, Prendergast M, Forman D and Cowley S. Outcome of pseudoseizures in children and adolescents: a 6-year symptom survival analysis. *Dev Med Child Neurol* 2001; **43**: 547–51.

27 Rutter N and Southall DP. Cardiac arrhythmias misdiagnosed as epilepsy. *Arch Dis Child* 1985; **60**: 54–6.

28 Commission on Classification and Terminology of the International League Against Epilepsy. Proposal for revised clinical and electro-encephalographic classification of epileptic seizures. *Epilepsia* 1981; **22**: 489–501.

29 Engel J. A proposed diagnostic scheme for people with epileptic seizures and with epilepsy: report of the ILAE Task Force on Classification and Terminology. *Epilepsia* 2001; **42**: 796–803.

30 Murdoch-Eaton D, Darowski M, Livingston J. Cerebral function monitoring in paediatric intensive care: useful features for predicting outcome. *Dev Med Child Neurol* 2001; **43**: 91–6.

31 Commission on Classification and Terminology of the International League Against Epilepsy. Proposal for classification of epilepsies and epileptic syndromes. *Epilepsia* 1989; **30**: 389–99.

32 Nordli DR, Bazil CW, Scheuer ML and Pedley TA. Recognition and classification of seizures in infants. *Epilepsia* 1997; **38**: 553–60.

33 Roger J, Bureau M, Dravet Ch, Genton P, Tassinari CA and Wolf P (eds). *Epileptic Syndromes in Infancy, Childhood and Adolescence*, 3rd edn. London: John Libbey, 2002.

34 Berg AT, Levy SR, Testa FM, Shinnar S. Classification of childhood epilepsy syndromes in newly diagnosed epilepsy: interrater agreement and reasons for disagreement. *Epilepsia* 1999: **40**: 439–44.

35 Berg AT, Shinnar S, Levy SR, Testa FM, Smith-Rapaport S and Beckerman B. How well can epilepsy syndromes be identified at diagnosis? A reassessment 2 years after initial diagnosis. *Epilepsia* 2000; **41:** 1269–75.

36 Baxter P, Griffiths P, Kelly T and Gardner-Medwin D. Pyridoxine dependent seizures: demographic, clinical, MRI and psychometric features, and effect of dose on intelligence quotient. *Dev Med Child Neurol* 1996; **38:** 998–1006.

37 Gordon N. Pyridoxine dependency: an update. *Dev Med Child Neurol* 1997; **39:** 63–5.

38 Appleton RE. Infantile spasms. *Arch Dis Child* 1993, **69:** 614–18.

39 Dulac O, Chugani HT and Dalla Bernardina B (eds). *Infantile Spasms and West Syndrome.* Philadelphia: WB Saunders, 1994.

40 Appleton RE. Landau–Kleffner syndrome. *Arch Dis Child* 1995; **72:** 386–7.

41 Singh R, Scheffer IE, Crossland K and Berkovic SF. Generalised epilepsy with febrile seizures plus: a common childhood-onset genetic epilepsy syndrome. *Ann Neurol* 1999; **45:** 75–81.

42 Tasch E, Cendes F, Li LM, Dubeau F, Andermann F and Arnold DL. Neuroimaging evidence of progressive neuronal loss and dysfunction in temporal lobe epilepsy. *Ann Neurol* 1999; **45:** 568–76.

43 Panayiotopoulos CP, Obeid T and Tahan AR. Juvenile myoclonic epilepsy; a 5-year prospective study. *Epilepsia* 1994; **135:** 285–96.

44 Scheffer IE, Bhatia KP, Lopes–Cendes I et al. Autosomal dominant nocturnal frontal lobe epilepsy: a distinctive clinical disorder. *Brain* 1995; **118:** 61–73.

45 Oldani A, Zucconi M, Ferini–Strambi L et al. Autosomal dominant nocturnal frontal lobe epilepsy: electroclinical picture. *Epilepsia* 1996; **37:** 964–76.

46 Ritaccio AL. *Reflex Epilepsies. Neurologic Clinics; Epilepsy II, Special Issues* (Volume 12). Philadelphia: WB Saunders, 1994; 57–83.

47 Binnie BD. Simple reflex epilepsies. In: Engel J and Pedley TA (eds). *Epilepsy: A Comprehensive Textbook.* Philadelphia: Lippincott-Raven, 1997; 2489–505.

48 Zifkin BG and Andermann F. Complex Reflex epilepsies. In: Engel J and Pedley TA (eds). *Epilepsy: A Comprehensive Textbook.* Philadelphia: Lippincott-Raven, 1997; 2507–13.

49 Fish DR, Quirk JA, Smith SJM et al. National survey of photosensitivity and seizures induced by electronic screen games (video games, console games, computer-games). Home and Leisure Accident Research Consumer Safety Unit, Department of Trade and Industry. London: HM Stationery Office, July 1994.

50 Quirk JA, Fish DR, Smith SJM et al. First seizures associated with playing electronic screen games: a community-based study in Great Britain. *Ann Neurol* 1995; **37:** 733–7.

51 Appleton R, Beirne M, Acomb B. Photosensitivity in juvenile myoclonic epilepsy. *Seizure* 2001; **9:** 108–11.

52 Ferrie CD, De Marco P, Grunewald RA et al. Video game-induced seizures. *J Neurol Neurosurg Psychiatry* 1994; **57:** 925–31.

53 Chadwick D, Cartlidge N and Bates D (eds). *Medical Neurology.* Edinburgh: Churchill-Livingstone, 1989.

54 Aicardi J. Epilepsy in brain-injured children. *Dev Med Child Neurol* 1990; **32:** 191–202.

55 Gibbs J and Appleton RE. The biochemical investigation of epilepsy in childhood. *Seizure* 1997; **6:** 193–200.

56 Gordon N. Epilepsy and disorders of neuronal migration. I: Introduction. *Dev Med Child Neurol* 1996; **38:** 1053–7.

57 Gordon N. Epilepsy and disorders of

neuronal migration. II: Epilepsy as a symptom of neuronal migration defects. *Dev Med Child Neurol* 1996; **38:** 1131 – 4.

58 Singh R, Gardner RJ, Crossland KM, Scheffer IE and Berkovic SF. Chromosomal abnormalities and epilepsy: A review for clinicians and gene hunters. *Epilepsia* 2002; **43:** 127–40.

59 Nordli DR Jr, De Vivo DC. Classification of infantile seizures: implications for identification and treatment of inborn errors of metabolism. *J Child Neurol* 2002; **17 (Suppl 3):** 3S3–3S8.

60 Buist NRM, Dulac O, Bottiglieri T et al. Metabolic evaluation of infantile epilepsy: summary recommendations of the Amalfi Group. *J Child Neurol* 2002; **17 (Suppl 3):** 3S98–3S102.

61 Rosman NP, Peterson DB, Kaye EM and Colton T. Seizures in bacterial meningitis: prevalence, patterns, pathogenesis and prognosis. *Pediatr Neurol* 1985; **1:** 278–85.

62 Annegers JF, Hauser WA, Beghi E, Nicolosi A and Kurland LT. The risk of unprovoked seizures after encephalitis and meningitis. *Neurology* 1988; **38:** 1407–10.

63 Golden GS. Pertussis vaccine and injury to the brain. *J Pediatr* 1990; **116:** 854–61.

64 Mustonen K, Mustakangas P, Uotila L, Muir P and Koskiniemi M. Viral infections in neonates with seizures. *J Perinat Med* 2003; **31:** 75–80.

65 Annegers JF, Grabow JD, Groover RV et al. Seizures after head trauma: a population study. *Neurology* 1980; **30:** 683–9.

66 Kieslich M and Jacoby G. Incidence and risk factors of post-traumatic epilepsy in childhood. *Lancet* 1995; **345:** 187.

67 Temkin NR, Haglung MM and Winn R. Causes, prevention and treatment of post-traumatic epilepsy. *New Horizons* 1995; **3:** 518–22.

68 Appleton RE and Demellweek C. Post-traumatic epilepsy in children requiring inpatient rehabilitation following head injury. *J Neurol Neurosurg Psychiatry* 2002; **72:** 669–72.

69 Schierhout G and Roberts I. Prophylactic antiepileptic agents after head injury: a systematic review. *J Neurol Neurosurg Psychiatry* 1998; **64:** 108–22.

70 Temkin NR, Dikman SS, Wilensky AJ et al. A randomised double-blind study of phenytoin for the prevention of post-traumatic seizures. *N Engl J Med* 1990; **323:** 497–502.

71 Iudice A and Murri L. Pharmacological prophylaxis of post-traumatic epilepsy. *Drugs* 2000; **59:** 1091–9.

72 Aicardi J. Epilepsies as a presenting manifestation of brain tumours and of other selected brain disorders. In: Aicardi J (ed). *Epilepsy in Children,* 2nd edn. New York: Raven Press, 1994; 334–53.

73 Patel H, Garg BP, Salanova V et al. Tumor-related epilepsy in children. *J Child Neurol* 2000; **15:** 141–45.

74 Ibrahim K and Appleton R. Seizures as the presenting symptom of brain tumours in children. *Seizure* 2003; (In press).

75 Cendes F, Andermann F, Dubeau F et al. Early childhood prolonged febrile convulsions, atrophy and sclerosis of mesial structures, and temporal lobe epilepsy: an MRI volumetric study. *Neurology* 1993; **43:** 1083–7.

76 Van Landingham KE, Heinz ER, Carazos JE et al. Magnetic resonance imaging evidence of hippocampal injury after prolonged focal febrile convulsions. *Ann Neurol* 1998; **43:** 413–26.

77 Cendes F, Cook MJ, Watson C et al. Frequency and characteristics of dual pathology in patients with lesional epilepsy. *Neurology* 1995; **45:** 2058–64.

78 Aksu F. Nature and prognosis of seizures in patients with cerebral palsy. *Dev Med Child Neurol* 1990; **32:** 661–8.

79 Carlsson M, Hagberg G and Olsson I. Clinical and aetiological aspects of epilepsy in children with cerebral palsy. *Dev Med Child Neurol* 2003; **45**: 371–6.

80 Hagberg B and Kyllerman M. Epidemiology of mental retardation – a Swedish survey. *Brain Dev* 1983; **5**: 441–9.

81 Besag F M. Childhood epilepsy in relation to mental handicap and behavioural disorders. *J Child Psychol Psychiatry* 2002: **43**: 103–31.

82 Robinson R and Gardiner RM. Genetics of childhood epilepsy. *Arch Dis Child* 2000; **82**: 121–5.

83 Bird TD. Genetic considerations in childhood epilepsy. *Epilepsia* 1987; **28 (Suppl 1):** S71–S81.

84 Greenberg DA, Durner M and Delgado-Escueta AV. Evidence for multiple gene loci in the expression of the common generalised epilepsies. *Neurology* 1992; **42 (Suppl 5):** 56–62.

85 Celesia GG. Are the epilepsies disorders of ion channels? *Lancet* 2003; **361:** 1238–9.

86 Blandfort M, Tsuboi T and Vogel F. Genetic counselling in the epilepsies. I: Genetic risks. *Hum Genet* 1987; **76:** 303–31.

87 Gardiner RM. Genetics. In: Wallace S (ed). *Epilepsy in Children*. London: Chapman and Hall Medical, 1996: 153–65.

88 Vigevano F and Fusco L. Hypnic tonic postural seizures in healthy children provide evidence for a partial epileptic syndrome of frontal lobe origin. *Epilepsia* 1993; **39:** 110–9.

89 Appleton RE, Farrell K, Applegarth DA et al. The high incidence of valproate hepatotoxicity in infants may relate to familial metabolic defects. *Can J Neurol Sci* 1990; **17:** 145–8.

90 Volpe JJ. Neonatal seizures. In: Volpe JJ (ed). *Neurology of the Newborn,* 3rd edn. Philadelphia: WB Saunders, 1995: 172–207.

91 Stafstrom CE. Neonatal seizures. *Pediatr Rev* 1995; **16:** 248–56.

92 Lombroso CT. Neonatal seizures: a clinician's overview. *Brain Dev* 1996; **18:** 1–28.

93 Evans D and Levene MI. Neonatal seizures. *Arch Dis Child Fetal Neonatal Ed* 1998; **78:** F70–F75.

94 Gordon N. Startle disease or hyperekplexia. *Dev Med Child Neurol* 1993; **35:** 1015–18.

95 Koning-Tijssen MA and Brouwer OF. Hyperekplexia in the first year of life. *Mov Disord* 2000; **15:** 1293–6.

96 Cokar O, Gelisse P, Livet MO et al. Startle response; epileptic or non-epileptic? The case for 'flash' SMA reflex seizures. *Epileptic Disord* 2001; **3:** 7–12.

97 Praveen V, Patole SK and Whitehall JS. Hyperekplexia in neonates. *Postgrad Med J* 2001; **77:** 570–2.

98 Zhon L, Chillag KL and Nigro MA. Hyperekplexia: a treatable neurogenetic disease. *Brain Dev.* 2002; **24:** 669–74.

99 Levene M. The clinical conundrum of neonatal seizures. *Arch Dis Child Fetal Neonatal Ed* 2002; **86:** F75–F77.

100 Goutieres F and Aicardi J. Atypical presentations of pyridoxine-dependent seizures. A treatable cause of intractable epilepsy in infants. *Ann Neurol* 1985; **17:** 117–20.

101 Hall RT, Hall FK and Daily DK. High-dose phenobarbital in term newborn infants with severe perinatal asphyxia: a randomised, prospective study with three-year follow-up. *J Pediatr* 1998; **132:** 345–8.

102 Boylan GB, Rennie JM, Pressler RM et al. Phenobarbitone, neonatal seizures, and video-EEG. *Arch Dis Child Fetal Neonatal Edition* 2002; **86:** F165–F170.

103 Painter MJ, Scher MS, Stein AD et al.

Phenobarbitone compared with phenytoin for the treatment of neonatal seizures. *N Engl J Med* 1999; **341:** 485–9.

104 Aicardi J. Febrile convulsions. In: Aicardi J (ed). *Epilepsy in Children*, 2nd edn. New York: Raven Press, 1994: 253–75.

105 Grunewald RA, Farrow T, Vaughan P, Rittey CD and Mundy J. A magnetic resonance study of complicated early childhood convulsions. *J Neurol Neurosurg Psychiatry* 2001; **71:** 638–42.

106 Ward N, Evanson J and Cockerell OC. Idiopathic familial temporal lobe epilepsy with febrile convulsions. *Seizure* 2002; **11:** 16–19.

107 Iwasaki N, Nakayama J, Hamano K, Matsui A and Arinami T. Molecular genetics of febrile seizures. *Epilepsia* 2002; **43 (Suppl 9):** 32–5.

108 Verity CM, Ross EM and Golding J. Outcome of childhood status epilepticus and lengthy febrile convulsions: findings of a national cohort study. *BMJ* 1993; **307:** 225–8.

109 Kuks JBM, Cook MJ, Fish Dr, Stevens JM and Shorvon SD. Hippocampal sclerosis in epilepsy and childhood febrile seizures. *Lancet* 1993; **342:** 1391–4.

110 Trinka E, Unterrainer J, Haberlandt E et al. Childhood febrile convulsions – Which factors determine the subsequent epilepsy syndrome? A retrospective study. *Epilepsy Res* 2002; **50:** 283–92.

111 Taikka R, Paakko E, Phytinen J, Uhari M and Rantala H. Febrile seizures and mesial temporal sclerosis: no association in a long-term follow-up study. *Neurology* 2003; **60:** 215–18.

112 Sutula TP. Progression in mesial temporal lobe epilepsy. *Ann Neurol* 1999; **45:** 553–5.

113 Chadwick D. Epilepsy continuing into adulthood. In: Wallace SJ (ed). *Epilepsy in Children* London: Chapman and Hall, 1996: 625–32.

114 Castle GF and Fishman LS. Seizures in adolescent medicine. *Paediatr Clin North Am* 1973; **20:** 819–35.

115 Cooper JE. Epilepsy in a longitudinal study of 5000 children. *Br Med J* 1965; **i:** 1020–2.

116 Janz D and Waltz S. Juvenile myoclonic epilepsy with absences. In: Duncan JS and Panayiotopoulos CP (eds). *Typical Absences and Related Epileptic Syndromes*. London: Churchill-Livingstone, 1994: 174–84.

117 Appleton RE, Chadwick DW and Sweeney A. Managing the teenager with epilepsy: paediatric to adult care. *Seizure* 1997; **6:** 27–30.

118 Appleton RE, Neville BGR. Teenagers with epilepsy. *Arch Dis Child* 1999; **81:** 76–9.

119 Sheth RD. Adolescent issues in epilepsy. *J Child Neurol* 2002; **17 (Suppl 2):** 2S23–2S27.

120 Dean JCS, Hailey H, Moore SJ et al. Long-term health and neurodevelopment in children exposed to antiepileptic drugs before birth. *J Med Genet* 2002; **39:** 251–9.

121 Crawford P. Epilepsy and pregnancy. *Seizure* 2001; **10:** 212–19.

122 Shorvon S. Antiepileptic drug therapy during pregnancy: the neurologist's perspective. *J Med Genet* 2002; **39:** 248–50.

123 Smith PEM. The teenager with epilepsy has special needs. *BMJ* 1998; **317:** 960–1.

124 Rowan AJ and French JA. The role of the encephalogram in the diagnosis and management of epilepsy. In: Pedley TA and Meldrum BS (eds). *Recent Advances in Epilepsy*. Edinburgh: Churchill-Livingstone, 1988: 63–92.

125 Carpay JO, de Ward AW, Schimisheimer RJ et al. The diagnostic yield of a second EEG after partial sleep deprivation: a prospective study in children with newly diagnosed seizures. *Epilepsia* 1997; **38:** 595–9.

126 Gibbs J, Appleton RE, Carty H, Beirne M and Acomb BA. Focal electro-encephalographic abnormalities and computerised tomography findings in children with seizures. *J Neurol Neurosurg Psychiatry* 1993; **56**: 369–71.

127 Cross JH, Jackson GD, Neville BGR et al. Early detection of abnormalities in partial epilepsy using magnetic resonance. *Arch Dis Child* 1993; **69**: 104–9.

128 Shinnar S, O'Dell C, Mitnick R, Berg AT and Moshe SL. Neuroimaging abnormalities in children with an apparent first unprovoked seizure. *Epilepsy Res* 2001; **43**: 261–9.

129 Harvey SA and Berkovic SF. Functional neuro-imaging with SPECT in children with partial epilepsy. *J Child Neurol* 1994; **9 (Suppl 1)**: S71–S81.

130 ILAE Neuroimaging Commission. ILAE Neuroimaging Commission recommendations for neuroimaging of patients with epilepsy. *Epilepsia* 1997; **38 (Suppl 10)**: 1–2.

131 Verity CM. When to start anticonvulsant treatment in childhood epilepsy: the case for early treatment. *BMJ* 1988; **297**: 1528–30.

132 Mellor D. When to start anticonvulsant treatment in childhood epilepsy: the case for avoiding or delaying treatment. *BMJ* 1988; **297**: 1529–30.

133 Shinnar S, Berg AT, Moshe SL et al. Risk of recurrence following a first unprovoked seizure in childhood: a prospective study. *Pediatrics* 1990; **85**: 1076–85.

134 Camfield C, Camfield P, Gordon K and Dooley J. Does the number of seizures before treatment influence ease of control or remission of childhood epilepsy? Not if the number is 10 or less. *Neurology* 1996; **46**: 41–4.

135 Appleton RE and The Mersey Region Paediatric Epilepsy Interest Group. Seizure-related injuries in children with newly diagnosed and untreated epilepsy. *Epilepsia* 2002; **43**: 764–7.

136 Wirrell EC, Camfield PR, Camfield CS, Dooley JM and Gordon KE. Accidental injury is a serious risk in children with typical absence epilepsy. *Arch Neurol* 1996; **53**: 929–32.

137 Verity CM, Hosking G and Easter DJ. A multicentre comparative trial of sodium valproate and carbamazepine in paediatric epilepsy. *Dev Med Child Neurol* 1995; **37**: 97–108.

138 Appleton RE. The treatment of infantile spasms by paediatric neurologists in the UK and Ireland. *Dev Med Child Neurol* 1996; **38**: 278–9.

139 Bobele GB and Bodensteiner JB. The treatment of infantile spasms by child neurologists. *J Child Neurol* 1994; **9**: 432–5.

140 Appleton RE, Peters ACB, Mumford JP and Shaw DE. Randomised, placebo-controlled study of vigabatrin as first-line treatment of infantile spasms. *Epilepsia* 1999; **40**: 1627–33.

141 Shinnar S, Vining EPG, Mellits ED et al. Discontinuing antiepileptic medication in children with epilepsy after two years without seizures. *N Engl J Med* 1985; **313**: 976–80.

142 Appleton RE. Withdrawal of long-term antiepileptic treatment in children. *Seizure* 1999; **8**: 381–3.

143 Peters AC, Brouwer OF, Geerts AT et al. Randomised prospective study of early discontinuation of antiepileptic drugs in children with epilepsy. *Neurology* 1998; **50**: 724–30.

144 Todt H. The late prognosis of epilepsy in childhood: results of a prospective follow-up study. *Epilepsia* 1984; **25**: 137–44.

145 Bouma PAD, Peters ACB and Brouwer OF. Long-term course of childhood epilepsy following relapse after antiepileptic drug withdrawal. *J Neurol Neurosurg Psychiatry* 2002; **72**: 507–10.

146 May W. Comments on EEG as a useful predictor of seizure recurrence after antiepileptic drug withdrawal in children. *J Epilepsy* 1991; **4:** 9–10.

147 Tennison M, Greenwood R, Lewis D and Thorn M. Discontinuing antiepileptic drugs in children with epilepsy. A comparison of a six week and a nine month taper. *N Engl J Med* 1994; **330:** 1407–10.

148 Dodson WE. Level off. *Neurology* 1989; **39:** 1009–10.

149 Appleton RE. Patient compliance. *BMJ* 1992; **305:** 1434.

150 Aicardi J. Surgical treatment. In: Aicardi J (ed). *Epilepsy in Children,* 2nd edn. New York: Raven Press, 1994: 429–39.

151 Snead 3rd OC. Surgical treatment of medically refractory epilepsy in childhood. *Brain Dev* 2001; **23:** 199–207.

152 Resnick TJ, Duchowny M and Jayakar P. Early surgery for epilepsy: redefining candidacy. *J Child Neurol* 1994; **9 (Suppl 2):** 2S36–2S41.

153 Duchowny MS. Surgery for intractable epilepsy: issues and outcome. *Pediatrics* 1989; **84:** 886–94.

154. Commission on Neurosurgery of the International League Against Epilepsy (ILAE) 1997–2001: Proposal for a new classification of outcome with respect to epileptic seizures following epilepsy surgery. *Epilepsia* 2001; **42:** 282–6.

155 Taylor DC. Callosal section for epilepsy and the avoidance of doing everything possible. *Dev Med Child Neurol* 1990; **32:** 267–70.

156 Berg AT and Vickrey BG. Outcome measures. In: Engel J Jr and Pedley TA, (eds). *Epilepsy: A Comprehensive Textbook.* Philadelphia: Lippincott-Raven, 1998: 1891–9.

157 Vagus Nerve Stimulation Study Group. A randomized controlled trial of chronic vagus nerve stimulation for treatment of medicinally intractable seizures. *Neurology* 1995; **45:** 224–30.

158 Hornig GW, Murphy JV, Schallert G and Tilton C. Left vagus nerve stimulation in children with refractory epilepsy: an update. *South Med J* 1997; **90:** 484–8.

159 Labar D. Vagus nerve stimulation for intractable epilepsy in children. *Dev Med Child Neurol* 2000; **42:** 496–9.

160 Boon P, Vonck K, De Reuck J and Caemaert J. Vagus nerve stimulation for refractory epilepsy: *Seizure* 2001; **10:** 448–55.

161 Prasad AN, Stafstrom CF and Holmes GL. Alternative epilepsy therapies: the ketogenic diet, immunoglobulins, and steroids. *Epilepsia* 1996; **37 (Suppl 1):** S81–S95.

162 Schwartz RH, Eaton J, Bower BD and Aynsley-Green A. Ketogenic diets in the treatment of epilepsy: short-term clinical effects. *Dev Med Child Neurol* 1989; **31:** 145–51.

163 Wheless JW. The ketogenic diet: fa(c)t or fiction. *J Child Neurol* 1995; **10:** 419–23.

164 Lefevre F and Aronson N. Ketogenic diet for the treatment of refractory epilepsy in children: a systematic review of efficacy. *Pediatrics* 2000; **105:** E46.

165 Hemingway C, Freeman JM, Pillas D and Pyzik PL. The ketogenic diet: a 3–6 year follow-up of 150 children enrolled prospectively. *Pediatrics* 2001; **108:** 898–905.

166 Kossoff EH, Pyzik PL, McGrogan JR, Vining EPG and Freeman JM. Efficacy of the ketogenic diet for infantile spasms. *Pediatrics* 2002; **109:** 780–3.

167 Egger J, Carter CM, Soothill JF and Wilson J. Oligoantigenic diet treatment of children with epilepsy and migraine. *J Pediatr* 1989; **114:** 51–8.

168 O'Regan ME and Brown JK. Is ACTH a key to understanding anticonvulsant action? *Dev Med Child Neurol* 1998; **40:** 82–9.

169 Gasior M, Carter RB, Goldberg SR and Witkin JM. Anticonvulsant and behavioral effects of neuroactive steroids alone and in conjunction with diazepam. *J Pharmacol Exp Ther* 1997; **282:** 543–53.

170 Snead OC, Benton JW and Myers GJ. ACTH and prednisolone in childhood seizure disorders. *Neurology* 1983; **33:** 966–70.

171 Hancock E, Osborne JP and Milner P. The treatment of West syndrome: a Cochrane review of the literature to December 2000. *Brain Dev* 2001; **23:** 624–34.

172 Van Engelen GBM, Renier WO, Weemaes CMR, Gabreels FJM and Meinardi H. Immunoglobulin treatment in epilepsy, a review of literature. *Epilepsy Res* 1994; **19:** 181–90.

173 Villani F and Avanzini G. The use of immunoglobulins in the treatment of human epilepsy. *Neurol Sci* 2002; **23 (Suppl 1):** S33–S37.

174 Mostofsky DI and Balaschak BA. Psychobiological control of seizures. *Psychol Bull* 1997; **84:** 723–50.

175 Ramaratnam S, Baker G A and Goldstein L. Psychological treatments for epilepsy *Cochrane Database Sys Rev* 2001: 4CD002029.

176 Wu D. Mechanism of acupuncture in suppressing epileptic seizures. *J Tradit Chin Med* 1992; **12:** 187–92.

177 Kloster R, Larsson P G, Lowssius R et al. The effect of acupuncture in chronic intractable epilepsy. *Seizure* 1999: **8:** 170–4.

178 Stavem K, Kloster R, Rossberg E et al. Acupuncture in intractable epilepsy: lack of effect on health-related quality of life. *Seizure* 2000; **9:** 422–6.

179 Pellock JM. Status epilepticus in children: update and review. *J Child Neurol* 1994; **9 (Suppl 2):** 2S27–2S35.

180 Mitchell WG. Status epilepticus and acute repetitive seizures in children,

adolescents and young adults: etiology, outcome and treatment. *Epilepsia* 1996; **37 (Suppl 1):** S74–S80.

181 Shorvon S. *Status Epilepticus. Its Clinical Features and Treatment in Children and Adults.* Cambridge: Cambridge University Press, 1994.

182 DeLorenzo RJ, Towne AR, Pellock JM and Ko D. Status epilepticus in children, adults and the elderly. *Epilepsia* 1992; **33 (Suppl 4):** S15–S25.

183 Lowenstein DH, Bleck T and Macdonald RL. It's time to revise the definition of status epilepticus. *Epilepsia* 1999; **40:** 120–2.

184 Emery ES. Status epilepticus secondary to breath-holding and pallid syncopal spells. *Neurology* 1990; **40:** 859.

185 Sillanpaa M and Shinnar S. Status epilepticus in a population-based cohort with childhood-onset epilepsy in Finland. *Ann Neurol* 2002; **52:** 303–10.

186 Maytal J, Shinnar S, Moshe SL and Alvarez LA. Low morbidity and mortality of status epilepticus in children. *Pediatrics* 1989; **83:** 323–31.

187 Shinnar S, Maytal J, Krasnoff L and Moshe SL. Recurrent status epilepticus in chlidren. *Ann Neurol* 1992; **31:** 598–604.

188 Advanced Life Support Group. Convulsions (status epilepticus). In: *Advanced Paediatric Life Support; the Practical Approach,* 2nd edn. London: BMJ Publishing Group 1997: 113–18.

189 The Status Epilepticus Working Party. The treatment of convulsive status epilepticus in children. *Arch Dis Child* 2000; **83:** 413–19.

190 Qureshi A, Wassmer E, Davies P, Berry K and Whitehouse WP. Comparative audit of intravenous lorazepam and diazepam in the emergency treatment of convulsive status epilepticus in children. *Seizure* 2002; **11:** 141–4.

191 Appleton RE, Sweeney A, Choonara I, Robson J and Molyneux E. Lorazepam vs

diazepam in the treatment of epileptic seizures and status epilepticus. *Dev Med Child Neurol* 1995; **37**: 682–8.

192 Yu KT, Mills S, Thompson N and Cuman C. Safety and efficacy of intravenous valproate in pediatric status epilepticus and acute repetitive seizures. *Epilepsia* 2003; **44**: 724–6.

193 Wallace SJ. Nasal benzodiazepines for management of acute childhood seizures? *Lancet* 1997; **349**: 222.

194 O'Regan ME, Brown JK and Clarke M. Nasal rather than rectal benzodiazepines in the management of acute childhood seizures. *Dev Med Child Neurol* 1996; **38**: 1037–45.

195 Kendall JL, Reynolds M and Goldberg R. Intranasal midazolam in patients with status epilepticus. *Ann Emerg Med* 1997; **29**: 415–17.

196 Kutlu No, Doğrul M, Yakinci C and Soylu H. Buccal midazolam for treatment of prolonged seizures in children. *Brain Dev* 2003; **25**: 275–8.

197 Browne TR. Fosphenytoin (Cerebyx). *Clin Neuropharmacology* 1997; **20**: 1–12.

198 Morton LD. Clinical experience with fosphenytoin in children. *J. Child Neurol* 1998; **13 (Suppl l)**: S19–S22.

199 Fischer JH, Patel TV and Fischer PA. Fosphenytoin: clinical pharmacokinetics and comparative advantages in the acute treatment of seizures. *Clin Pharmacokinet* 2003; **42**: 33–58.

200 Appleton RE and Gill A. Adverse events associated with intravenous phenytoin in children: a prospective study. *Seizure* 2003; **12**: 369–72.

201 O'Donohoe NV. What should the child with epilepsy be allowed to do? *Arch Dis Child* 1983; **58**: 934–7.

202 Carpay HA, Vermeulen J, Stroink H et al. Disability due to restrictions in childhood epilepsy. *Dev Med Child Neurol* 1997; **39**: 521–6.

203 Kemp AN and Silbert JR. Epilepsy in children and the risk of drowning. *Arch Dis Child* 1993; **68**: 684–5.

204 Bazil CW. Sleep-related epilepsy. *Curr Neurol Neurosci Rep* 2003; **3**: 167–72.

205 Krumholz A. Driving and epilepsy: a historical perspective and review of current regulations. *Epilepsia* 1994; **35**: 668–74.

206 Kokkonen J, Kokkonen E-R, Saukkonen A-L and Pennanen P. Psychosocial outcome of young adults with epilepsy in childhood. *J Neurol Neurosurg Psychiatry* 1997; **62**: 265–8.

207 Hoare P. The development of psychiatric disorder among schoolchildren with epilepsy. *Dev Med Child Neurol* 1984; **26**: 3–13.

208 Hoare P. Psychiatric disturbances in the families of epileptic children. *Dev Med Child Neurol* 1984; **26**: 14–19.

209 Holdsworth L and Whitemore K. A study of children with epilepsy attending normal schools. I: Their seizure patterns, progress and behaviour in school. *Dev Med Child Neurol* 1974; **16**: 746–58.

210 Schoenfeld J, Seidenberg M, Woodard A et al. Neurophysiological and behavioural status of children with complex partial seizures. *Dev Med Child Neurol* 1999; **41**: 724–31.

211 Kwan P and Brodie MJ. Neuropsychological effects of epilepsy and anti-epileptic drugs. *Lancet* 2001; **357**: 216–22.

212 Austin JK, Harezlak J, Dunn DW, Huster GA, Rose DF and Ambrosius WT. Behaviour problems in children before first recognised seizures. *Pediatrics* 2001; **107**: 115–22.

213 Baker GA, Hesdon B and Marson AG. Quality-of-life and behavioral outcome measures in randomized controlled trials of anti-epileptic drugs: a systematic review of methodology and reporting standards. *Epilepsia* 2000; **41**: 1357–63.

214 Stores G. School children with epilepsy at

risk for learning and behaviour disorders. *Dev Med Child Neurol* 1978; **20**: 502–8.

215 Besag FMC. Epilepsy, education and the role of mental handicap. *Ballieres Clin Paed* 1994; **2**: 561–83.

216 Bannon MJ, Wildig C and Jones PW. Teachers' perceptions of epilepsy. *Arch Dis Child* 1992; **67**: 1467–71.

217 Tidman L, Saravanan K and Gibbs J. Epilepsy in mainstream and special education primary school settings. *Seizure* 2003; **12**: 47–51.

218 Scott RC, Besag FM and Neville BGR. Buccal Midazolam and rectal Diazepam for treatment of prolonged seizures in childhood and adolescence; a randomised trial. *Lancet* 1999; **353**: 623–6.

219 Morrow JI. Specialised epilepsy clinics – the pros and cons. *Seizure* 1993; **2**: 267–8.

220 Cunningham C, Newton R, Appleton R, Hosking G and McKinlay I. Epilepsy – giving the diagnosis. A survey of British paediatric neurologists. *Seizure* 2002; **11**: 500–11.

221 Appleton RE and Sweeney A. The management of epilepsy in children: the role of the clinical nurse specialist. *Seizure* 1995; **4**: 287–91.

222 Risdale I, Kwan I and Cryer C. Newly diagnosed epilepsy: can a nurse specialist help? A randomized controlled trial. Epilepsy Care Evaluation Group. *Epilepsia* 2000; **41**: 1014–19.

223 Bradley P and Lindsay B. Specialist nurses for treating epilepsy. *Cochrane Database Sys Rev* 2001; 4CD001907.

224 Brown S, Betts T, Chadwick D et al. An epilepsy needs document. *Seizure* 1993; **2**: 91–103.

225 Kitson A, Shorvon S. Clinical Standards Advisory Group. *Services for Patients with Epilepsy*. London: Department of Health, 2000.

Index

Italic page numbers refer to the drugs directory on pages 108 to 118.